Kurz

Textbook of Dr. Vodder's
Manual Lymph Drainage

Volume 2: Therapy

# Textbook of Dr. Vodder's Manual Lymph Drainage

Volume 2: Therapy

By Ingrid Kurz MD
Preface by Emil Vodder Ph. D. †

Translated by
Robert H. Harris HND (Appl. Biol. U.K.)

With 16 illustrations

4th edition

**Karl F. Haug Verlag · Heidelberg**

**Die Deutsche Bibliothek – CIP-Einheitsaufnahme**

**Textbook of Dr. Vodder's manual lymph drainage.** – Heidelberg : Haug
Dt. Ausg. u. d. T.: Lehrbuch der manuellen Lymphdrainage nach Dr. Vodder
Früher u. d. T.: Introduction to D[octo]r Vodder's manual lymph drainage

Vol. 2. Therapy / by Ingrid Kurz. Transl. by Robert H. Harris. Pref. by Emil
Vodder. – 4. ed. – 1997
ISBN 3-7760-1671-X

1st edition 1986 – 3rd edition 1993

© 1997 by Karl F. Haug Verlag, Hüthig GmbH, Heidelberg

ISBN 3-7760-1671-X

Production: Progressdruck, 67346 Speyer, Germany

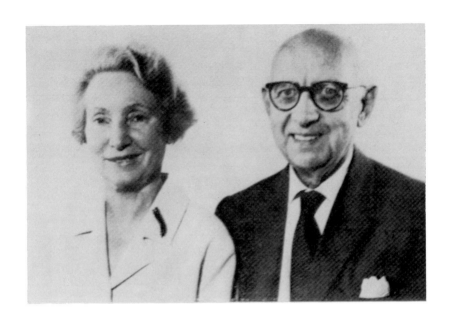

*Respectfully and gratefully dedicated to
Dr. Emil Vodder † and Estrid Vodder †,
the founders of Manual Lymph Drainage*

## Translator's Note

This book was translated by *Robert H. Harris* HND, (Appl. Biol., U.K.), who is a registered massage therapist in Toronto, Canada, and specializes in manual lymph drainage therapy.
He would especially like to thank *Christine Donald*, M.A. (Cantab.), for her excellent criticism and assistance in correcting the translated work. His thanks go also to *Pauli Schell* for typing the text.

Toronto, Canada, April 1986

## Please pay attention:

We would like to point out to the reader that the term "lymph capillary" is increasingly being replaced by the term "initial lymph vessel". As this change in the nomenclature of lymphology is not accomplished yet, we have decided to apply the "old" term in the present new edition.

# Contents

## Preface by Dr. phil. Emil Vodder

Now that this present book about Manual Lymph Drainage by Dr. *Ingrid Kurz* is available, we have the first medical textbook of our lymph drainage method.

Whereas Volume I deals primarily with the practice, here we find the theoretical basis carefully and thoroughly compiled. Without this, a new method cannot be accepted. We are particularly grateful that Dr. *Ingrid Kurz* has built upon and deepened her extensive knowledge through many years of practical work in this area.

It is particularly significant for us that our intuitively conceived method has now been scientifically explained in such a profound way after years of practical success.

We hope this book will disclose much understanding to the readers as far as practical work is concerned also.

Frau Dr. *Ingrid Kurz* deserves great thanks for this considerable achievement. Our best wishes go with her in her future work.

Kopenhagen-Bagsvaerd, 26. 1. 1979

Dr. *Emil Vodder* †

# Preface by the Author

In 1971 Dr. *Emil Vodder* and *Estrid Vodder* began to teach Manual Lymph Drainage (M.L.D.) to massage therapists and aestheticians in Walchsee, in the school named after them. The training for massage therapists, health professionals and aestheticians developed from these week-long basic courses.

In the beginning, the therapeutic application of M.L.D. was tested on various types of indications by a handful of doctors (Dr. *Asdonk,* Dr. *Westphal,* Dr. *Stricker* to name a few). Based upon these experiences, the possible therapeutic uses of M.L.D. expanded.

Faced with a new mode of treatment, orthodox medicine was, to say the least, cautious, if not even disapproving. It wanted to see scientific evidence for the effectiveness of the *Vodder's* method. So in the period following, Prof. *Földi* and Prof. *Mislin* provided proof, as far as lymphology was concerned, of the way that M.L.D. works and its effectiveness.

This was the blueprint for the theoretical teaching material at the Dr.-Vodder-School in Walchsee. The teaching plan at that time developed from the experiences collected during the courses.

The theoretical classes of the therapy course require a knowledge of human anatomy, histology, and physiology, as imparted by the massage schools.

A special knowledge of lymphology and blood capillary physiology is necessary in order to explain the action of M.L.D. Therefore the fundamental principles of this special area of anatomy and physiology are briefly reviewed in this book.

Volume 3 offers the areas of indication for M.L.D. The individual symptoms are discussed as well as the way M.L.D. is used with the respective illnesses and an explanation of the effects of M.L.D. in each of these indications. The therapist must know about the illness and its cause in order that M.L.D. can be adapted to the particular symptoms. She/he should know how M.L.D. works and what results to expect.

The subject matter of both these therapy volumes corresponds to the present level of technical knowledge, so far as the literature and lectures are available. Neither volume claims to be complete.

The compilation of symptoms suitable for treatment with M.L.D. is based on many years of experience in the application of this method. Presumably in the next few years more areas of indication will be added. I already know of individual cases successfully treated with M.L.D., which are from these inadequately proven areas of indication. If these results are obtained in sufficient numbers with similar illnesses, then the catalogue of indications for M.L.D. can be expanded.

Walchsee, January 1979

# Introduction

Dr. *Vodder's* M.L.D. achieves its effect in the body in various ways. It acts:

I   on oedema reduction
 1. through the lymphatic system
 2. through the blood capillaries
 3. the lymph-obligatory load is shunted from oedemous tissue over watersheds to regions with a functioning lymphatic system

II   on the nervous system
 1. on the autonomic system
 2. by reducing pain

III   on the muscular system
 1. on skeletal muscle
 2. on vessel wall muscle
 3. on peristalsis

IV   on the immune system

The Vodder manual technique has its own characteristics which are decisive for the effect of M.L.D.:

a) pumping: smooth pressure increase and decrease with no pressure in the zero phase
b) circular movements or spirals
c) with close skin contact, movement of the skin over the underlying tissues
d) in the direction of lymph flow. At first the proximal area is treated, distal to proximal, then in the same manner moving progressively distal
e) rhythmic
f) painless

ad.I   All six criteria of the manual technique must be observed exactly for an oedema reducing effect. The oedema fluid behaves like an inert mass. It can be shunted through the tissue with steadily increasing, but not excessively strong pressure. This effect is supported by the pumping (increasing and decreasing pressure), the circular hand movement and the rhythm of the movement sequence. The degree of pressure must be adapted to the oedema and is relatively small in relation to other classical massage techniques. Of similar importance is the "freeing" of proximal lymph vessels for the drainage of lymph moved from distal areas. M.L.D. must be painless, as pain can increase the oedema.

ad.II   The effect on the autonomic system is particularly influenced by the rhythmic succession of movements. The circular, pumping sequence of movements supports the effect.

ad.II   Stroking the touch receptors in the subcutis is particularly important for the analgesic effect. Attention must be paid to exert the correct amount of pressure, as well as to the rhythmic and painless application.

ad.III  The correct pressure, rhythm and painless application are all important for the effect on the muscular system.

ad.IV   Experience teaches us that the body's defence system is favourably affected by M.L.D. The following hypothetical explanation suggests itself: pathogens reach the lymph nodes through the lymphatic system, where antibodies are formed. These go into circulation via the lymph system. Therefore good lymph circulation can distribute the antibodies quickly.

# A) The Blood-Vessel System

The blood vessels, together with the heart as a pump, form a closed vessel system. The blood which travels through this vessel system transports $O_2$ and nutrients to the tissues, and $CO_2$ and metabolic products back from the tissues. Blood also has the function of distributing hormones and various active substances within the body.

# 1. Structure of the Vessels

### a) Aorta

The aorta and large arteries are supplied with an INTIMA (endothelial cell layer), under which lies the ELASTICA INTERNA. In the small arteries this layer merges into the basal lamina, as is found in the capillaries. The MEDIA is a layer of smooth muscle cells, which can be very pronounced in some arteries. Surrounding this is the ELASTICA EXTERNA and the ADVENTITIA borders on this. This forms the connection to the surrounding connective tissue. The elastic wall construction of the aorta makes the "ripple effect" possible (continuous blood movement during systole and diastole).

### b) Arteriole

The precapillary arteries are described as ARTERIOLES and have a very strong media consisting of muscles cells lying in circles. With these "precapillary sphincters" they regulate capillary flow. In some organs the METARTERIOLE also occurs between the arteriole and capillary. It does not have an enclosed muscle layer, but rather muscles cells that go in circles, and this enables the metarteriole to func-

17

tion as a sphincter. With their strongly muscular media, the arterioles regulate the blood supply in their capillary area. They are the vessels of resistance in the circulation. If a precapillary sphincter closes completely, the blood runs directly through the ARTERIOVENOUS ANASTOMOSIS into the veniole.

The CAPILLARY NETWORK begins after the arteriole or metarteriole sphincters. It is an extensive network supplied by one or several arterioles. In some organs, as for example the brain, retina and heart, small arteries have no collaterals (parallel paths to the mainstream, in this case the arteries): the capillary network is only supplied by one arteriole, the end-artery. If an embolus or thrombus blocks the blood vessel, the tissue supplied by the capillary becomes necrotic ( = tissue decay).

### c) Vein

The first part of the venous vessel segment is called the VENIOLE (venule), which continues from the venous capillary network. The VEIN wall is also constructed in three layers. The muscle layer is essentially weaker than in the arteries and the veins have VALVES, which are important for the blood-flow back to the heart since they determine the direction of the flow. A functional disturbance of these valves plays a role in the formation of venous leg oedema.

### d) Capillary

The CAPILLARY WALL consists solely of an ENDOTHELIAL CELL LAYER and the basal membrane underneath. This BASAL MEMBRANE consists of thinly woven reticulum fibrils with small pores between their mesh which have a diameter of 30—70 Ångstrom (1 Ångstrom = $10^{-10}$m). [18] Between these collagen fibrils lies an amorphus ground substance. In many organs the capillary basal lamina splits into two parts surrounding a paricyte. On the inside the pericyte is in direct contact with the endothelial cells; on the outside the basal membrane covers it. [18] The pericyte probably plays a role in the construction of the basal membrane. It contains many small pinocytotic vacuoles, which indicate that substances are transported through the cells. The size and thickness of the pores in the basal membrane determine what substances can pass through the membrane, and in what quantity.

However the connection between endothelial cells is also decisive here. These cells can lie closely together, as for example in the muscle, lungs or brain, but they can also have an intracellular opening, as in the intestinal villi or in the kidneys. In the liver, the endothelial cells have an intercellular gap formation and no basal membrane.

Diffusion and filtration through a capillary wall are not only determined by diameter, the degree of blood pressure in this region and the colloid-osmotic pressure relationship, but also by the structure of the capillary wall (type of endothelial cell, thickness and pore size of the basal membrane). [18] In the brain, for example, the blood capillaries have a particularly thick basal membrane, and nourishment of the ganglion cell (organ cell) occurs via the glia cell rather than by diffusion.

The CAPILLARIES are 0.5 − 1mm long and their diameter can vary between 4 and 10 μm. The capillary can also change its diameter, probably through changes in the shape and size of the endothelial cell. Since the capillary diameter can be smaller than that of the erythrocytes (7 μm), the erythrocytes can become distorted when passing through the capillary, and they then lie like pointed caps lengthwise beside each other. A gush of plasma follows this roll of erythrocytes before the next erythrocyte clump, mostly led by a granulocyte, is pushed through the capillary. Therefore the flexibility of the erythrocyte also plays a role in capillary circulation and thus also in tissue nourishment. A certain minimum blood pressure is also necessary to push the erythrocyte group through the capillaries.

Water and small molecular substances can leave the capillary between the endothelial cells. Also large molecular substances — such as protein — can leave the vessel lumen via MICROPINOCYTOSIS. During micropinocytosis (where protein is concerned, the process is also called CYTOPEMPSIS), a part of the endothelial cell membrane surrounds a protein molecule in the bloodstream enclosing it in an envelope of cell membrane and passing it as a vesicle through the cell.

19

On the endothelial cell the vesicle opens, the envelope is taken up by the cell membrane and its contents — the protein — lie outside the blood vessel in the surrounding tissue. This process can happen in the venous capillary network, but occurs particularly often in the venioles.

Within 24 hours, approximately $50 - 100$ % of the plasma proteins leave the bloodstream in this way and are taken via the lymph vessel system as lymph-obligatory load back to the venous system. [3] Histamine and other vessel-effective substances (such as those that appear during inflammation) dilate the blood capillary wall and increase its permeability not only for water and small molecular substances, but also for large molecular substances such as protein. This process is of great significance in the formation of inflammatory and allergic oedemas.

The CIRCULATION OF THE CAPILLARY NETWORK is controlled by the arterioles but also affected by signals coming from the metabolic processes in the pericapillary tissue. Thus a drop in pressure of $O_2$ or rise of $CO_2$ content has a relaxing effect on the sphincters of the arterioles as does an acidic pH change. A temperature increase also widens the arterioles. The effect of histamine has already been mentioned. To some extent the regulation of circulation in the capillary area occurs independently of blood pressure regulation in the arterial circulation. Thus, frequently, an arterial hypertonia is connected with a decreased blood supply in the capillary area. Congestion in the venous network can raise the pressure in the capillary area and subsequently increase the filtration.

# 2. Nutrition and Nervous Supply of the Circulatory System

The inner layers of the vessel wall are nourished by diffusion, whereas the adventitia has nutrient vessels, the "VASA VASORUM" (artery, vein, lymph vessel), entering the vessel wall. The nervous supply of the blood vessels occurs through the AUTONOMIC NERVOUS SYSTEM (sympathetic, parasympathetic): the blood vessels' muscular system is supplied by the SYMPATHETIC nerves, and stimulation produces vasoconstriction (narrowing of vessels). This causes a blood pressure increase in vessels which produce peripherial resistance. Vasodilation occurs as a result of excitation of the parasympathetic system only in skeletal muscle. In all other vessels vasodilation happens through a decrease of the sympathetic tonus. [22]

The filling condition of the capillaries and arteries is inferred by skin colour and temperature: the amount of blood, which is regulated by the arteriole, determines skin temperature, whereas the capillary filling gives the skin its colour. Thus in cold conditions the skin is pale and cool, since capillaries and arterioles are narrowed. During warmth, the skin is reddened and warm as the capillaries and arterioles are opened. If the skin is pale (narrow capillaries) and warm (dilated arterioles), heat congestion is indicated, as seen during heat stroke. Blueish-red, cold skin is a sign of dilated capillaries and narrow arterioles, as seen with frost-bite. [22]

Blood capillaries are capable of REGENERATION. They appear in scar tissue and a real vascularisation occurs. The body can also balance a nutritional deficiency ($O_2$-deficiency) in the tissues through an improved capillarisation (capillary hypertrophy, as seen during height adaption in alpine regions). [23]

# 3. Regulation of Blood Pressure and Flow

The regulation of blood pressure occurs through complex processes: the autonomic nervous system, hormones such as angiotensin, cortisone, adlosterone or the enzyme renin and also through ions. It is generally known that an increased supply of sodium chloride in the diet, for example, can lead to an increased blood pressure. The quantity of blood flowing through a cross section of the aorta and the opened capillaries within a time period is equal. Since the sum total of the capillary diameters is 1 000 times larger than that of the aorta, blood flows 1 000 times faster in the aorta than the capillaries. The exchange of substances important for all nutrition occurs through the walls of these slow flowing capillaries. Because of the unequal pressure during systole and diastole, blood flow in the aorta and large vessels varies in speed. [22]

Flow speed, blood pressure and diameter of the vessel play an important role in cell nutrition. They follow circumscribed physical laws.

Circulation is regulated by changes in the vessel radius, and the body can also regulate the filling of various capillary areas. Part of the blood volume is stored in the venous system, in the spleen and the liver. The capillaries are never all open at the same time. Blood distribution is oriented towards nutritional needs (work output).

# 4. Blood

The blood consists of cells — the blood cells — and plasma. Its volume is approximately 5.6 litres in adults. The ERYTHROCYTES, red blood cells, are formed in the bone marrow and enter the blood as nucleus-free, round, disc-shaped cells. They are approximately 2 μm thick and 7.5 μm in diameter. Their life span is about 120 days. Men have approximately 5 million erythrocytes and women 4.5 million. They are carriers of haemoglobin, which transports oxygen. They cannot move of their own accord but are pushed along with the bloodplasma.

The white blood cells, LEUCOCYTES (approx. 4 000—8 000 in healthy adults), only spend a part of their life span in the blood and remain much longer in the bone marrow, the lymphatic or connective tissue. These include:

- Granulocytes: neutrophils, eosinophils
- Lymphocytes
- Plasma cells
- Monocytes

NEUTROPHILIC GRANULOCYTES: $8-14\,\mu m$ large, have amoeboid movement and originate in the bone marrow. Their granula contains enzymes, which are capable of phagocytosis ("eating", e.g. bacteria). They belong to the microphages. Each cell only lives approximately 30 hours. They are attracted by bacteria or general inflammatory processes in the body (chemotaxis), and they leave the circulation ("police" of the body) through the vessel walls. During inflammatory diseases they are to be found in the blood in increased numbers (leucocytosis). Approximately $55-68\,\%$ neutrophilic granulocytes occur in the normal white blood count.

BASOPHILIC GRANULOCYTES: somewhat larger than the neutrophils, their cell body is rich in histamine and heparin (anti-clotting substance). They are similar to mast cells (according to differing views, either identical or related). Their portion of the white blood count varies between 0.5 and 1 %.

ESINOPHILIC GRANULOCYTES: $2-3\,\%$ of the white blood count, increasing during allergies. They are capable of taking up the antigen-antibody complex (see immunology) and breaking it down. This is why an increase is shown in the tissues and blood during allergic reactions.

LYMPHOCYTES: $20-35\,\%$ of the white blood count, with a diameter of $6-8\,\mu m$. There are long lived lymphocytes (memory cells of the immune system, with a life span of up to one year) and short lived ones (life span of a few days). They have many functions during the various immune reactions and are formed in the bone marrow and all lymphatic organs (spleen, thymus, and lymph nodes). There are large and small lymphocytes, whose differing size should indicate their activity level. We differentiate between B- and T-lymphocytes according to their immunological functions. Their variable form is only recognizable under the electron microscope — not the light microscope. The white blood count contains increased lymphocytes during chronic inflammation.

PLASMA CELLS: their portion in the blood is under 1 %. They are found in rich supply in the lymph nodes and in the tissue. Their

23

cell is oval and the nucleus the same as that in the lymphocytes. There are vacuoles in their protoplasm containing gamma globulin which is given up to the blood plasma (see: Immunology).

MONOCYTES: diameter 15 − 20 µm. Formed in the bone marrow. They have amoeboid movement, belong to the reticulohistiocytary system and are macrophages. They can also phagocytose cells or cell debris. According to many authors, they are the preliminary stage of histiocytes (tissue macrophages). [13]

THROMBOCYTES: (blood platelets), 2 − 4 µm. Their mother cells (megacariocytes) are formed in the bone marrow. An important factor in blood clotting, they contain serotonin, which causes vasoconstriction and helps stop bleeding during injuries.

BLOOD PLASMA: contains ions, dissolved inorganic and organic molecules. Albumin and globulin form the larger part of plasma proteins (blood protein, about 7 − 7.4 %). Through electophoresis (movement of charged colloid particles in an electric field), the various fractions of albumin and globulin can be differentiated. The plasma proteins move at different speeds in the electric field.

The ALBUMINS are long, oval molecules (38 Å crosswise and 150 Å lengthwise) and are thus able to leave the vessel walls more easily than the round globulin molecules (185 Å diameter). Albumins are formed in the liver and function (in the blood) as carriers (e.g. for hormones). Like all plasma proteins, they provide an oncotic suction in the blood through their water binding capability.

The balance between albumin and globulin shifts — in favour of globulin — during inflammatory illness. This shift increases the BLOOD SEDIMENTATION RATE, and thus an increased sedimentation indicates an inflammatory illness. There are also other causes for an increased blood sedimentation.

The plasma cells provide GAMMA-GLOBULINS to the blood. They are the active substance of humoral immunity.

FIBRINOGEN: plays a role in blood clotting and is also contained in the lymph.

Besides the plasma proteins, blood also contains ORGANIC and INORGANIC SUBSTANCES: [22]
- inorganic ions (electrolytes): Ca, Cl, Fe, Cu, Mg, K, Na, phosphate, bicarbonate, iodine.

24

● organic component: fats, (lipids, to which cholesterol and trigly-cerides belong), lipoproteins (fat/protein-combinations), glucose (elevated values in diabetes), lactic acid (increased during oxygen deficient metabolism), pyruvic acid, enzymes, hormones, vitamins, ketone bodies, nitrogen-containing bonds (partly metabolic build-ing blocks such as amino acids, partly breakdown products such as substances normally contained in the urine like urea, uric acid) and bile pigments.

## 5. Physiology of the Blood Capillaries

The Starling-Hypothesis deals with the relationship of hydrostatic with colloid-osmotic pressure in the area of blood capillaries. The interaction of these forces decides whether a balance of fluid-exchanges will develop in the capillary bed, whether an increased flow of fluid will continue into the tissue which can then be taken away by the lymph system, or whether an oedema will develop. Impulses come also from the tissue and these influence capillary flow via the arterioles (regulation through the arteriole musculature): from metabolites (from cell metabolism in the surrounding tissues), from the autonomic system, changes in the permeability of the capillary wall through histamine and other "tissue hormones" and reactions to tactile perception. Therefore the regulation of processes at the capillary is subject to many influences. STARLING himself did not use numbers for his model, because the conditions at the capillary are different in various tissues.

In order to understand these processes, some physical concepts need to be explained:

### a) Filtration

Filtration is a process, in which fluid is forced through a membrane as a result of the hydrostatic pressure difference on both sides of the membrane. The amount of filtrate is dependent on the nature of the filter area and the pressure difference. [22] The capillary wall has the characteristics of a semi-permeable (semi-porous) membrane, and fluid and small molecular substances are pushed through it into the pericapillary tissue by the force of blood pressure. Blood corpuscles and large molecular components of the blood remain in the vessel lumen. The amount of filtrate is dependent on the surface area and permeability of the capillary wall, on the capillary blood pressure and also on the strength of forces counteracting this filtration (colloid-osmotic pressure of plasma proteins, tissue pressure). On average the daily volume of filtrate in the body reaches 70 litres. This is of minor significance in volume, compared with diffusion. Filtration occurs at a transcellular as well as an intercellular level.

## b) Diffusion

Diffusion is described as the thorough mixing of solutions of various concentrations through their thermal energy.

THERMAL MOLECULAR MOVEMENT is the motor of diffusion. The constantly moving particles of a solution (a gas mixture) collide, bounce off each other and thus, in time, are fully mixed together. A temperature increase speeds up particle movement. (No movement at absolute zero, $-273.15\,°C$.)

The SIZE OF THE PARTICLES is also important: the smaller the particles, the faster the movement. The TIME OF DIFFUSION increases with the square of distance. Diffusion as a transport mechanism is therefore only suitable over short distances. The daily volume of diffusion in the body lies between 20 000—60 000 litres.

The exchange of substances between capillary and cell follows the principles of diffusion through the capillary wall and the ground substance. A disturbance in this environment, which extends the DIFFUSION DISTANCE, e.g. in oedema formation, delays CELL NUTRITION by the SQUARE OF THE DISTANCE. The condition of the basal membrane of the capillary plays a large role in diffusion.

26

## c) Osmosis

In osmosis, we are concerned with diffusion through a semi-permeable membrane. On one side of the membrane is a dissolved substance which cannot pass through the pores of the membrane. The solvent, which is also on the other side of the membrane, can diffuse through the membrane pores in both directions. Consequently an equilibrium appears: equal numbers of solvent molecules form on both sides of the membrane as a result of the diffusion through the membrane. In addition, however, there are still on the one side the molecules of the substance which cannot diffuse through the membrane pores because of their size. On this side the total solution volume will be higher than the side containing only solvent. Depending on which side of the membrane the pressure-effect is viewed, one may speak either of an OSMOTIC PRESSURE or of an OSMOTIC SUCTION. ONCOTIC SUCTION is understood as an osmotic (or also colloid-osmotic) suction from proteins. This oncotic suction of blood proteins contributes appreciably in the equilibrium as a counterbalance to blood pressure.

## d) The Starling Equilibrium

At the turn of the century, *Starling* observed a regularity in fluid movement at the blood capillary. As a result of the hydrostatic pressure of the blood pressure, fluid escapes through the semi-permeable wall of the blood capillary into the surrounding tissue (capillary bed). The suction of the plasma proteins counteracts this filtration force of plasma proteins in the blood stream. The relation between filtration (fluid movement into peri-capillary tissue) and resorption (entry of fluid into the blood capillary from the interstitium) shifts according to the construction of the capillary wall and blood pressure. In addition, a decreased content of plasma protein in the blood capillary changes the relationship of filtration to resorption.

*Földi* [3] utilized these expressions: effective filtration pressure and effective colloid-osmotic pressure.

Accordingly:
effective filtration pressure = capillary blood pressure — tissue pressure
effective colloid-osmotic pressure = blood colloid-osmotic pressure — tissue colloid-osmotic pressure.

But also, the size of these two measurements, effective filtration pressure and effective colloid-osmotic pressure, depends on the capillary wall construction, its permeability, its length and also on the respective arterial and venous capillary loops. Taking all these factors into consideration, it is clear that fluid movements of varying strength occur in the various bodily tissues. This is due not only to the differing construction of the blood capillary wall, but also to the differing capillary circulation depending on the operative condition of the tissue. [29]

How can an INCREASED FILTRATION occur in the tissue?

1. The B.P. can INCREASE IN THE CAPILLARY. There are various causes. The most significant one is a back flow from the venous system. Other causes: reactive, after previous compression or lack of blood, by enlargement of the capillary lumen, through nutritional deficiency in the surrounding tissue with accumulation of metabolites, through the effects of histamine, application of heat and through the autonomic nervous system.

2. During conditions of PROTEIN DEFICIENCY: If the plasma proteins decrease, the osmotic pressure in the blood falls. Therefore resorption at the venous loop is also smaller.

3. An INCREASED PERMEABILITY of the capillary wall can occur: under the effect of histamine or other substances which appear during tissue inflammation, through medicines and chemical substances.

As soon as effective filtration pressure is greater than effective colloid-osmotic pressure, this excess amount of fluid becomes lymph-obligatory load: the LYMPH-TIME-VOLUME (amount of lymph in a time unit) increases.

# 6. Oedema-Reducing Effect of Manual Lymph Drainage (M.L.D.)

The oedema-reducing effect of Dr. *Vodder's* M.L.D. takes place in many various ways. Experiments indicate that mild tactile stimulations, such as the special manual technique of M.L.D., activate the lymph motoricity. M.L.D. is of special importance when lymph motoricity is excited in the normal area bordering on lymph-oedomatous areas. With lymphostatic, protein-rich oedemas, the lymph-obligatory load is shunted further into the tissue spaces until areas are reached where the lymph transport (still) functions. In addition, increased resorption of excess tissue fluid can occur over the venous capillary loop.

The massage pressure of M.L.D. depends, on the one hand, on the type of tissue being worked on and, on the other, the nature of the oedema. The massage pressure is therefore not uniform but varies from case to case. For healthy ("normal") tissue and slight oedema the guide line is that no reddening of the skin should occur through M.L.D. if it is applied correctly. An exception to this rule is patients with positive (= red) dermatography where, basically, one must always work with less pressure (although a slight reddening cannot be avoided in every case).

When considering the tissues, the thickness and nature of the individual skin layers, especially the subcutaneous layer, play an important role — as does the turgor of the skin. Thus the treatment of an atrophic, loose, aged skin, for example, calls for less massage pressure than an eutrophic, youthful skin. Also the given or intended massage pressure depends proportionately on what lies beneath the skin: cartilage (or perichondrium), bones (or periosteum), tendon, aponeurosis, ligament, muscles or muscle fascia. In the last, most frequent case, muscle tone also plays an important role. The manual technique must be suited to the part of the body being worked on: one must consider whether the massage pressure can spread sideways or be fully effective in the area treated, as in the circular technique. Incidentally, the massage pressure is guided by the nature of the prevailing oedema: circumference and tension ("hardness") of the oedema, as well as its special characteristics: sol-gel relationship, protein and fibrous content ("degree of fibrosis") etc.

Diagnostically and therapeutically, it is now clear that the massage therapist needs expert use of touch, learned by experience. This is absolutely necessary for successful M.L.D. treatment — as it is for massage in general.

# B) The Connective Tissue

Every massage technique that works through the skin on the underlying tissues works on, for example, fluid, which lies in the subcutis. But not only this. It also works simultaneously on all the tissue structures in the subcutis — on blood vessels, lymph vessels, nerves and especially on the autonomic pathways, just as much as, for example, the sweat glands. Many massage techniques pay too little attention to regulation via the autonomic pathways.

The blood capillaries are situated in the connective tissue and filtration and diffusion take place through their walls. If fluid remains as oedema, this too takes place in the connective tissue. This group of tissues has very varied functions and correspondingly differing manifestations. It is recognised as true SUPPORT TISSUE in bones and cartilage. The original sense of the term "connective tissue" is that it CONNECTS TISSUE GROUPS and separates organs from their surroundings. As a RESERVOIR, it receives salts, vitamins, fat and water. The ground substance contains a great deal of water and is thus important for the WATER BALANCE. The fat content of the connective tissue and regulation of circulation play a role in BALANCE OF WARMTH. The connective tissue is CAPABLE OF REGENERATION: where organ tissues perish, and where a loss of volume occurs in the tissues, fibroblasts multiply and fill the defect with cells, fibres and ground substance. Capillaries also grow into this area. Connective tissue also serves as a DEFENCE mechanism: on one hand, the weave of its fibres forms a mechanical obstacle; on the other, there are many micro- and macrophages which destroy intruders, e.g. bacteria, through phagocytosis. However some of the pathogens can also contain enzymes which dissolve parts of the connective tissue (pneumococci and streptococci contain hyaluronidase, an enzyme that breaks down hyaluronic acid; also Clostridium bacilli produce collagenase, with which they can dissolve the collagen fibres;). [9]

*Pischinger* differentiates three forms of connective tissue: [12]
1. the cell-rich mesenchyme (corresponds to embryonal connective tissue)
2. fibre-rich connective and fat tissue
3. taut and hard connective tissue (tendons, ligaments, cartilage and bone)

ad.2. Loose, amorphous, soft, connective tissue belongs to this group, in which blood and lymph pathways lie, and through which exchange of substances between capillaries and cells takes place (interstitium). Therefore an oedema could be formed here. Cells of the reticulohistiocytary system are active here.

What are the components of connective tissue?
1. Cells
   a) fixed cells
   b) mobile cells
2. Fibres
   a) collagen fibres
   b) reticulin fibres
   c) elastic fibres
3. Ground substance
4. Fat tissue

## 1. Cells

### a) Fixed Cells

These are the connective tissue cells or fibrocytes. Here the fibro-blast is important, a substantially more active "mother" of the fibro-cytes. The environment of the connective tissue is regulated by these cells and they ensure the continued existence of cells through their multiplication. They grow into organ defects and there they form the scar tissue. Ground substance and the 3 fibril types originate in the body of these cells and are then deposited in their surroundings. The formation of tropocollagen can be increased in the cell by means of a mechanical effect. This collagen-precursor moves from the cell in a soluble form, the molecules aggregate and collagen fibrils are formed in the immediate vicinity of the cell.

### b) Mobile Cells

The MAST CELL occurs everywhere in loose connective tissue. Above all, it is found in the immediate vicinity of vessels. Like the basophilic granulocytes of the blood, these cells have much heparin-bound histamine in their granules. If an inflammation occurs in the tissues, this HISTAMINE comes out of the mast cell; it causes a dilation and increased permeability of the small vessels, stimulates the pain receptors in the tissue and probably takes part in attracting granulocytes to the damaged tissue. In addition it effects a vasoconstriction of the large vessels, [14] bronchospasm, colic in the intestinal region, and urticarial skin symptoms with itching. Mast cells can carry antibodies (Ig E). If however an antigen-antibody reaction occurs, histamine is set free from the mast cell, the symptom of which is known as an ALLERGIC reaction. This mechanism can play a large role in allergic bronchial asthma, just as in allergic skin eczemas. It is thus important for the therapeutic use of M.L.D. not to set off these mechanisms which worsen the symptoms.

NEUTROPHILIC GRANULOCYTES: they are active as microphages, which increase during inflammatory reactions in the tissue. They are found as an embankment around haematoma and work to take away the blood escaping into the tissue; also they are found in increased numbers in tissue changed by oedema.

LYMPHOCYTES: these appear in increased numbers where immunological reactions occur in the tissues. Greater numbers are found in the tissues during the course of the body's reaction to oedema formation. [19]

PLASMA CELLS: Similarly, these are found in the connective tissue during immunological tissue reactions.

HISTIOCYTES: these belong to the reticulohystiocytary system. In the shape of the nucleus and protoplasm, this cell closely resembles the blood monocyte. However the cell is usually not round, but irregular in shape. Some authors view them as monocytes migrating into the tissues, where they adapt to the prevailing conditions through a change in shape. [13] Other authors view them as individual cell types, closely related to monocytes. The histiocyte is an important tissue macrophage. It appears more frequently in newly formed oedema. [19] As long as there are many histiocytes in oedematous tissue, a proteolytic breakdown of proteins occurs. The small molecular components can then be taken away by the venous loop of the blood capillaries. It has been observed that, in the presence of cumarines and similar pharmaceutical substances, proteolysis in the tissue increases. [20] Therefore these preparations are given as support in oedema treatment with M.L.D. We were able to establish that, where there are lymphostatic oedemas, pathways form along the connective tissue fibres. The lymph-obligatory load follows these towards functioning lymph pathways. These fissures in the tissues can be covered with cells which look like endothelial cells and possibly originate from histiocytes.

ESINOPHILIC GRANULOCYTES: they increase during allergic reactions in the tissue because they have the ability to take up and break down antigen-antibody complexes.

# 2. Fibres

## a) Collagen Fibres

STRUCTURE: The tropocollagen molecules formed from the fibroblasts consist of three braided polypeptide chains of 1 000 amino acids wound together. [21] These lie together end-to-end and side-by-side. These pro-collagen filaments are then connected in pairs to protofibrils. The MICROFIBRIL is composed of several protofibrils and has a characteristic diagonal striping. Meshed FILAMENTS lie inside these microfibrils in an amorphous GROUND SUBSTANCE. This ground substance gives collagen fibrils their flexibility. The fibril is covered by a netlike tube, so that the ground substance, which has a lubricating effect, cannot be squeezed out of the fibril network by the effect of tension. As a 4th layer, the collagen fibril has another ring structure which prevents its being snapped off. [9]

PROPERTIES AND OCCURENCE: Because of this structure the collagen fibres are a high tensile element. They stretch very little (5%) and are well suited for power transmission. Therefore they are found in the body everywhere transference of tension or particular strain occurs: in bones, cartilage, tendons, fascia and in the subcutis. In addition, they are found with elastic fibres in the body where they have a MODERATING FUNCTION. When stretched, the elastic fibre is as long as the collagen fibre lying next to it. In this way elastic fibres can only be stretched to the length of the collagen fibres and are thus protected from overstretching or tearing.

## b) Reticulin Fibres

They provide the basic mechanical framework of the RETICU-LAR CONNECTIVE TISSUE. They occur in many organ tissues (liver, kidneys) as the connection to parenchyma cells, as well as in loose connective tissue. They form felt-like entanglements in the basal membranes. They are made from similar material to collagen fibres but are considerably finer.

## c) Elastic Fibres

Like both other types of fibres, these are also formed by the fibroblasts. Elastic fibres always occur as a net. They consist of elastin that has partly similar, partly dissimilar constituents to collagen. They are subject to an ageing process whereby their elasticity declines greatly.

If an elastic system is stretched over a long period of time, it cannot return to its original length when the tension is relieved. A residual stretching remains. This is also a reason why a drained oedematous arm does not usually regain its original circumference, but remains larger.

OCCURENCE OF THE ELASTIC FIBRE NETWORK: in the skin, arteries, lungs, elastic cartilage and the connective tissue capsules of various organs. In skin the ageing process of elastic fibres leads to wrinkles. Pregnancy stretch-marks (striae gravidarum) appear when the elastic and collagen-fibre network stretches and tears. The rippling effect of the aorta is caused by a particularly large proportion of elastic network in its wall. The ageing process and overstretching of the elastic network in the lungs leads to emphysema.

# 3. Ground Substance

Ground substance is formed in the fibroblasts. It contains water, electrolytes, amino acids, peptides as well as hormones, vitamins and various proteins. It is the course of transit for the migration of these substances from capillary to cell. PROTEINS are found in a liquid form (Sol) in the ground substance. However they are also bound in the PROTEOGLYCANES (acidic mucopolysaccharides, hyaluronic acid). GLYCOPROTEINS also contain protein. Above all, they occur in the basal lamina. Just like proteins, MUCOPOLYSAC-CHARIDES have a strong waterbinding capacity. They are viscous and in a gel state in the ground substance. The enzyme HYALU-RONIDASE breaks down HYALURONIC ACID and thereby liquefies the ground substance. Hyaluronic acid is also the bonding substance, by means of which the filaments are fixed to the endothelial cells of the lymph capillary wall. That is why hyaluronidase damages the tensile strength of these filaments, causing inadequacy in the opening mechanism of the lymph capillary. Bacteria that contain hyaluronidase liquefy the ground substance.

THIXOTROPHY: [21] ground substance can behave thixotrophically. This process is observed in the viscosity of the synovia. During warmth and strong movement, it becomes liquid. If the joint fluid is at a standstill for several hours and in somewhat lower temperatures (e.g. during sleep at nigth), the viscosity increases: the macromolecules of the ground substance aggregate into network structures. With warmth and movement, these aggregates dissolve again. This aggregation of macromolecules is known as thixotrophy. If heavy pressure is very suddenly applied, the connective tissue can show a brittle consistency and corresponding tendency to tear. (The macromolecules do not have time to orientate themselves spacially.) This is why tendon and muscle tears occur in sport when no appropriate warm-up is employed beforehand. (Sports massage before competitive sport.) A tear of the achilles tendon is typical when competing in cold conditions without a warm up. Tendon and muscle tears occur particularly often during sudden unexpected application of force.

*Pischinger* [12] interprets the cell-environment-complex as a functional unit. He defines under that heading the connective tissue lying between the organ cells, together with connective tissue cells, ground substance, blood and lymph capillaries, leucocytes, monocytes and individual cells where the parasympathetic and sympathetic nerve pathways terminate. A network of free axons comes from here, which lies directly in the ground substance of the connective tissue. The

38

connective tissue, with its physical and colloid-chemical changes, would thus be connected to the connective tissue in all other areas of the body, through the autonomic nervous system. PISCHINGER'S SYSTEM OF BASIC REGULATION thus provides an explanation of the long distance effect of M.L.D. which can be observed repeatedly during therapy.

In practice: we can treat one side because the other is in too much pain or in a plaster cast preventing treatment. If only one ulcer of a large, two sided ulcera cruris was treated with M.L.D., the rate of healing after this treatment would be significantly improved in the ulcers of both legs. When dealing with scar tissue, extensive additional work is carried out on healthy areas of the skin.

# 4. Fatty Tissue

This is a form of connective tissue. The fat exists in the cell as liquid droplets, and the cell nucleus and protoplasm are at the edges of the cell. The fat cells are fixed in their environment through a combination of elastic and collagen fibres. Thus they shift under the influence of pressure and return to their old position when the pressure ist released. [9]

FUNCTION: as a FAT LAYER on the palm of the hand, sole of the foot, buttocks, orbit, cheek and renal bed. In a fasting state this is broken down only after the storage fat.

As STORAGE FAT: subcutis, greater omentum under the peritoneum of the colon. Surplus calories (joules) are stored as fat and they resupply the body's metabolism during nutritional deficiency. The sub-cutaneous fat layer helps to protect the body temperature from cooling off.

# C) The Lymphatic System

# Summary

The blood vessel system has a closed circulation. The lymphatic system however begins blind in the tissues with its capillaries. The lymph angiones are strung together to form lymph vessels. Several of these vessels respectively lead to an intermediate lymph node from which one or two vessels proceed. Collector lymph nodes are frequently interposed before the large main lymph vessels join with the venous system in the right or left venous arch. The VENOUS ARCH (ANGULUS VENOSUS) develops from the confluence of the jugular (neck) and subclavian (arm) veins; Dr. *Vodder* calls this the TERMINUS in his instructions for treatment. The course of the lymph vessels show diverse variations considerably more often than the blood vessels.

There is a lack of lymph capillaries in cartilage, nails, epidermis, in the brain and spinal cord, in the inside of the eye, in all epithelial tissue and in the epithelial parenchyma of the large glands. Likewise, they are missing in parenchyma consisting of lymphoreticular mesenchyma cells; therefore they are absent in the spleen, bone marrow and lymphatic tissue; also in undifferentiated, taut connective tissue, e.g. that in the Dura mater. [1]

It is very important to know the position of the lymph vessels, because the order of movements in M.L.D. is orientated to their course. The therapist must also know where the large collector lymph nodes are and the anastomoses between individual lymph drainage areas (position of the "watersheds").

The superficial drainage areas of the body are divided according to the median sagittal plane (right and left halves of the body) (Figs.1 and 2). Numerous anastomoses (connections) exist between both drainage areas along this dividing line. However the transitions between other drainage areas of the body also show substantial anastomoses. Apart from this, there are connections in some lymph nodes between in and out flowing lymph vessels that consequently bypass the lymph nodes.

There are two LYMPH CAPILLARY NETWORKS in the SKIN. The superficial one lies in the Corium near the superficial arterial capillary network. This lymph capillary network is mostly without valves and is connected to the 2nd deeper network. This lat-

43

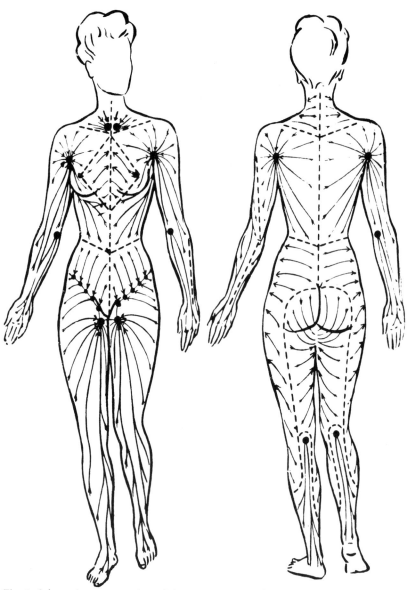

Fig. 1: Schematic representation of the body's lymph drainage of the skin (anterior), with the collecting lymph nodes: "terminus", axillary lymph nodes, inguinal lymph nodes. (Dr. *Vodder* [25])

Fig. 2: Schematic representation of the body's superficial lymph drainage pathways (posterior) (Dr. *Vodder* [25])

ter is in the corium beneath the deep arterial capillary network. The efferent vessels from this deep lymph capillary network begin with valves. They lead to SUBCUTANEOUS LYMPH VESSELS which are connected among themselves with anastomoses in a NET-LIKE manner. The lymph capillary networks are very pronounced at places which are exposed to strong pressure, e.g. the sole of the foot. [1] The efferent lymph vessels (CONDUCTING VESSELS) consist of lymph angiones and therefore have numerous valves, but still no coherent musculature. They lead into the COLLECTING VESSELS which now have the complete structure of lymph angiones with valves and circular muscle (28). They lie in the subcutis and, on their way to the collecting lymph nodes, have many cross connections to parallel lymph vessels. The course and anastomoses in these epifascial pathways are often decisive as to what extent oedema appears during a traumatic disruption of the main lymph vessels.

The lymph vessels of the musculature of the extremities proceed sub-fascially and flow into the deep lymph vessels, which follow the long bones and go to their respective collecting lymph nodes. These lymph vessels lie mostly in the immediate vicinity of arteries and veins.

# 1. Lymph Drainage Pathways of the Body

### a) Lower Extremity

Lymph from the subcutis of the SOLE of the FOOT and CALF, together with the lymph vessels from the calf musculature drain to the INTERMEDIATE NODES behind the KNEE. A collector vessel goes from there along the femur to the deep (inguinal) lymph nodes of the groin. Lymph from the DORSAL SKIN OF THE FOOT, the front of the LEG and from the THIGH is drawn to the INGUINAL lymph nodes. There is a group of lymph nodes in the adductor canal which are connected to the inguinal lymph nodes. Lymph from the skin around the anus and inner side of the thigh ("saddle" of the thigh) is taken over the inner side of the thigh to the inguinal lymph nodes. From the skin of the LOWER ABDOMEN and the buttocks up to an imaginary line from the navel, over the iliac crest (Crista iliaca) to the mid lumbar vertebrae, the lymph flows likewise to the inguinal lymph nodes. The lymph vessels of the outer genital skin also empty there.

### b) True Pelvis

From the INGUINAL LYMPH NODES the lymph vessels go alongside the femoral artery and vein, under the inguinal ligament into the inner pelvis. Here they proceed along the Linea terminalis division between true and false pelvis adjacent to the iliac artery and vein to the FORK OF THE AORTA. In this area the lymph vessel frequently divides into several cross-connected branches, interrupted by many lymph nodes. Lymph from the urogenital organs of the true pelvis also joins at this point: from the urethra, bladder, ureter, from the prostate in men, from the uterus and ovaries in women. These vessels also pass trough lymph nodes on the floor of the pelvis or on the side walls of the true pelvis. Lymph from the anus and rectum goes to the iliosacral lymph nodes (these lie on the inner side of the sacrum) and from there to the nodes in the fork of the aorta.

### c) Abdomen

These lymph vessels go from the fork of the aorta upwards to the cisterna chyli lying next to the vena cava inferior as the TRUNCUS LUMBALIS DEXTER, or next to the aorta as the TRUNCUS LUMBALIS SINISTER. There are also many intermediate lymph nodes here. Often we are dealing here, not with a truncus, but with a network of lymph vessels ("lymphatic plexus"). On their way, these vessels receive lymph from the organs of the large (false) pelvis: from the paired organs: URETER, KIDNEYS and ADRENALS. Lymph from the SPLEEN, PANCREAS, STOMACH, DUODENUM, GALL BLADDER and the under surface of the LIVER goes to the Truncus coeliacus. This belongs, as does the Truncus intestinalis, together with the lymph from the INTESTINAL FOLDS, to the catchment area of the Cisterna chili. There are many lymph nodes interposed between the organ and the main lymphatic trunk (very numerous in the mesentery!). The name, Cysterna chyli, comes from the lymph of the small intestine, which contains emulsified fat and is known as Chylus. The lymph from the convex side of the liver and the liver capsule flows in its lymph vessels through the diaphragm to the mediastinal and sternal lymph nodes. It joins with the Ductus lymphaticus dexter in the right venous arch.

Lymph from the muscular abdominal wall empties into both Trunci lumbales. The Cisterna chyli lies next to and behind the aorta at the level of the 2nd lumbar to the 12th thoracic vertebra. Not only can there be a great variation in the height of its position between these levels, but it can also be completely absent.

### d) Inner Thorax

The THORACIC DUCT (see Fig. 3 and 4), is the largest lymph vessel. It begins with the Cysterna chyli or the confluence of the Trunci lumbales and intestinalis. It ascends together with the aorta (lying to its right and dorsal) through the aortic opening in the diaphragm. In the posterior mediastinum it ascends vertically to the right of the aorta, close to the spinal column. Behind the aortic arch it turns to the left in front of the 5th thoracic vertebra, upwards along the spinal column to the left of the oesophagus. Opposite the 7th cervical vertebra it turns forward in order to join the left venous arch. It receives the Trunci jugularis, subclavius and bronchomediastinalis, just before this junction, or else these main branches join separately or in a different order.

In its thoracic course, the THORACIC DUCT ("thoracic milk pathway") receives the INTERCOSTAL LYMPH VESSELS which pass through lymph nodes in the intercostal spaces and usually also those beside the spinal column. Lymph from the lower intercostal lymph vessels is brought by the Trunci intercostales descendes dexter and sinister (descending lymph vessels of the R and L intercostal spaces) through the diaphragm to the thoracic duct or Cysterna chyli (Fig. 5). The intercostal lymph vessels are connected with the parasternal vessels (lateral to the sternum), whose lymph flows to the ter-

47

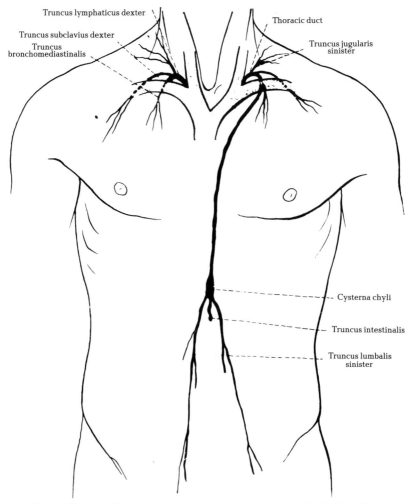

Truncus lymphaticus dexter

Thoracic duct

Truncus subclavius dexter

Truncus
bronchomediastinalis

Truncus jugularis
sinister

Cysterna chyli

Truncus intestinalis

Truncus lumbalis
sinister

Fig. 3: Diagram of the course of the large lymphatic trunks *(J. Tandler* [26])

minus (Fig. 6). In addition, numerous anastomoses in the intercostal spaces go to the vessels of the musculature and skin via the thorax. Thus, through the intercostal lymph vessels, connections exist between the catchment area of the thoracic duct in the thorax and the parasternal lymph vessels, which flow into the venous arch of the same side.

48

In the thorax, three lymphatic trunks on the right and three on the left collect the lymph from its organs and inner wall: the TRUNCUS BRONCHOMEDIASTINALIS, TRUNCUS PARASTERNALIS, TRUNCUS MEDIASTINALIS ANTERIOR. The Trunci broncho-mediastinales collect the lymph from the nodes at the side of the aorta and oesophagus as well as from the lungs and numerous lymph nodes in the mediastinum. The left Truncus bronchomediastinalis chiefly takes lymph from the upper left lobe of the lung. Lymph from the lower left lobe and the heart is directed together with lymph from the right lung to the right Truncus bronchomediastinalis. [1] According-ing to other authors [24], anastomoses frequently occur in the medias-tinum between lymph vessels from the organs in the right and left path of the thorax. The thoracic duct receives the left Trunci medias-tinalis anterior and parasternalis. The right Truncus mediastinalis anterior flows either directly into the venous arch or, like the Trun-cus parasternalis, first into the Truncus bronchomediastinalis, then together with this into the DUCTUS LYMPHATICUS DEXTER. This large lymph trunk originates from the confluence of the right Trunci jugularis, subclavius and bronchomediastinalis. It can be miss-ing if these 3 vessels flow directly into the Angulus venosus dexter. The Ductus lymphaticus dexter is usually only a few centimeters long before it leads into the right venous arch.

### e) Outer Thorax and Upper Extremity

The MAIN COLLECTING LYMPH NODES of the upper extremity lie in the AXILLA of the same side. Lymph of the OUTER THORAX wall also flows there. The division of drainage between the left and right axilla occurs on the rear side along the spinous proc-esses and on the front side from the jugular fossa to the navel. As mentioned previously, the border with the inguinal catchment area is from the navel, over the iliac crest to the mid lumbar vertebra. The upper, dorsal border of the area draining directly to the "terminus" is the spine of the scapula and the upper ventral border is the clavicle. The lymph drainage of the front side of the thorax, including both breasts, has an unusual feature. If the MAMMARY GLANDS are

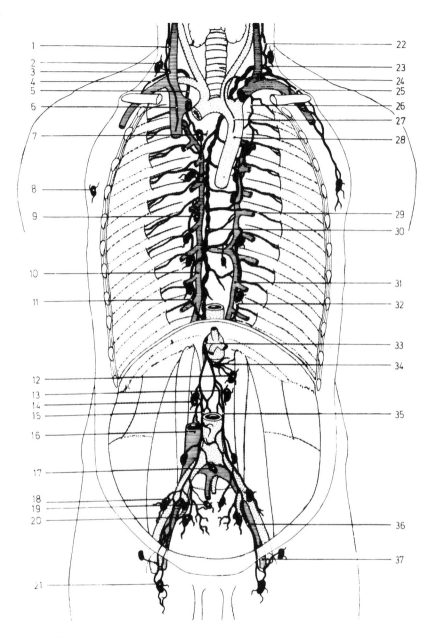

Fig. 4: Diagram of the main lymph trunks and their junction in the venous system and large lymph nodes (*Wenzel*, changed according to *Kampmeier* [5])

1 = Truncus jugularis (right)
2 = Deep cervical lymph nodes
3 = Junction of the Truncus jugularis dexter in the Angulus venosus
4 = Truncus subclavius (right)
5 = Truncus bronchomediastinalis (right)
6 = Truncus mediastinalis anterior (right)
7 = Lymph nodes in the mediastinum
8 = Axillary lymph nodes
9 = Intercostal lymph nodes
10 = Azygos vein
11 = Truncus lymphaticus intercostalis descendens (right)
12 = Mesenteric lymph nodes
13 = Lymph nodes on the aorta
14 = Lumbar lymph nodes
15 = Truncus lumbalis (right)
16 = Vena cava inferior
17 = Lymph nodes on the fork of the aorta
18—20 = Lymph nodes of the true pelvis
21 = Inguinal lymph nodes
22 = Truncus jugularis (left)
23 = Thoracic duct
24 = Junction of the thoracic duct
25 = Truncus subclavius (left)
26 = Truncus bronchomediastinalis (left)
27 = Truncus mediastinalis anterior (left)
28 = Aorta
29 = Intercostal lymph pathways
30 = Thoracic duct
31 = Hemiazygos vein
32 = Truncus lymphaticus intercostalis descendens (left)
33 = Cisterna chyli
34 = Truncus intestinalis
35 = Truncus lumbalis (left)
36 = Lymph vessels beside iliac artery and vein (Truncus lymphaticus iliaci)
37 = Femoral vein

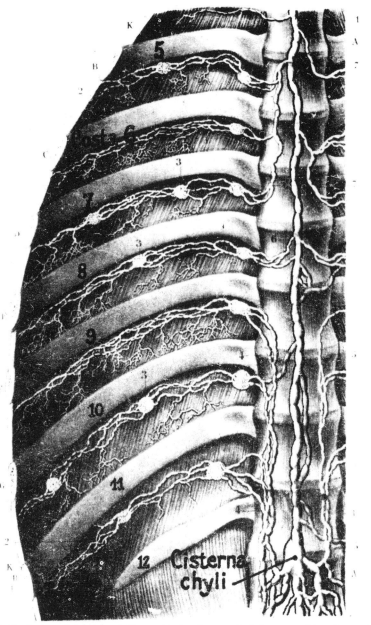

Fig. 5: Beginning of the thoracic duct with the cisterna chyli. Intercostal lymph vessels and intercostal nodes. Truncus lymphaticus descendens dexter and sinister (descending thoracic vessels according to *Vodder*[25])

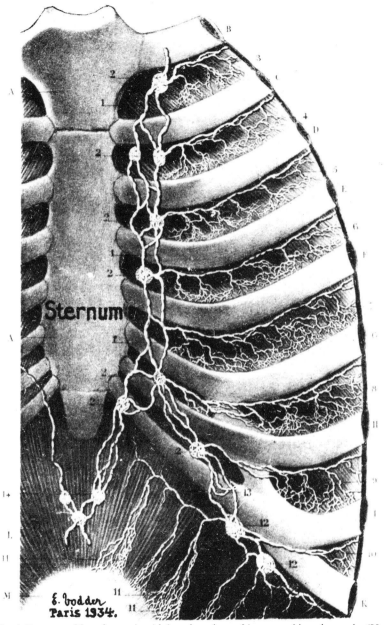

Fig. 6: Parasternal lymph vessels with lymph nodes and intercostal lymph vessels. *(Vodder*[25]*)*

divided into 4 quadrants, then the lymph of both lateral quadrants drains to the axilla. The medial upperquadrant drains to the subclavicular lymph nodes and then to the terminus. Lymph from the medial lower quadrant flows parasternally (next to the sternum) into the intercostal space and on the inner thorax wall along the costal arch to the spinal column then into the thoracic duct (Fig. 1, 5, 6, 7).

The LYMPH VESSELS OF THE ARM have intermediate lymph nodes in the elbow, in the medial bicipital groove, and flow into the collector lymph nodes of the axilla. Lymph from the skin above the ball of the shoulder (above the deltoid muscle) flows directly to the terminus (Fig. 7).

Lymph from the arm musculature flows subfascially to the large lymph vessels along the humerus, which also goes to the axillary lymph nodes. The Truncus subclavius connects the axillary lymph nodes to the terminus of the same side.

Occasionally, lymph vessels of the arm show variations in their course, which can be important after mastectomy. There are numerous anastomoses between parallel lymph pathways in the subcutis of the arm. Frequently the pathways from the radial catchment area (from thumb and index finger) do not go to the axillary lymph nodes, but rather along the cephalic vein, via the subclavicular lymph nodes, directly to the venous arch.

The Ductus lymphaticus dexter which consists of the Trunci bronchomediastinalis, subclavius and jugularis flows into the RIGHT ANGULUS VENOSUS.

The thoracic duct with lymph from both legs, organs of the true and false pelvis, and from the catchment area of the Trunci bronchomediastinalis, subclavius and jugularis sinister, flows into the LEFT ANGULUS VENOSUS.

## f) Head and Neck

Lymph from the skin and musculature of the head and neck is brought by the TRUNCUS JUGULARIS on each side to the venous arch on the same side. The lymph nodes of the neck region are particulary numerous and lie superficially, as well as deep in the tissues. There is no strict division between right and left drainage and there

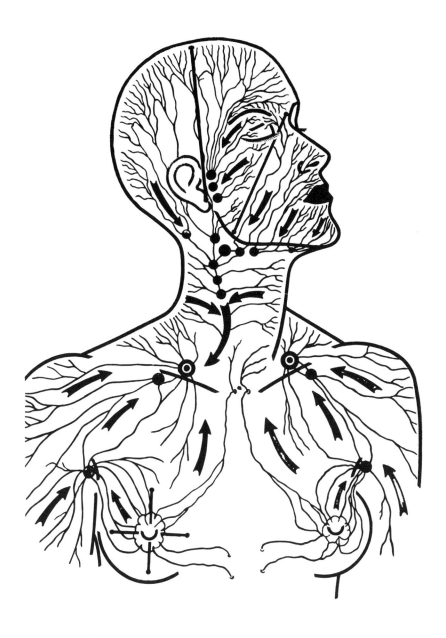

Fig. 7: Diagram of the lymph drainage from the head, neck and breast (4 quadrants) and from over the shoulder directly to the terminus. *(Vodder* [25])

55

are many connections to the opposite side. Numerous lymph nodes lie next to the nasopharynx, trachea, oesophagus and thyroid gland. In addition the lymph-obligatory load of the brain flows through the neck lymph vessels and the superficial and deep lymph node chains (Fig. 7).

### g) Anastomoses between the Various Lymph Drainage Areas

Some of the anastomoses (WATERSHEDS) are particularly important in the treatment of oedema. Those of therapeutic importance should be mentioned here.

The watershed between the catchment areas of the inguinal and that of the axillary lymph nodes lies in the middle of the body, i.e. from the navel, over the iliac crest to the mid-lumbar vertebrae. If, for example, the lymph drainage pathways in the inguinal lymph node region are interrupted, then the lymph-obligatory load is shunted over the watershed to the catchment area of the axillary lymph nodes. Besides this, paravertebral drainage is possible into the deep lumbar region to the para-aortal lymph vessels in the abdominal cavity and consequently to the Cysterna chyli and thoracic duct. Physiological anastomoses occur between the lymph vessels of the ceiling of the abdomen and inner wall of the abdominal cavity. In the thorax, the intercostal, paravertebral and parasternal anastomoses, especially, are available for therapeutic use. The axillary catchment area is connected through them to the thoracic duct. In case of a unilateral obstruction of the lymph drainage, connections to the opposite side over the sternum and spinous processes can be used in therapy. The lymph vessels in the arm have a connection between the axillary catchment area and that of the terminus in the skin over the deltoid muscle of the upper arm. Similarly, there are anastomoses between axillary and terminus lymph vessels over the clavicle and scapula. In the head-neck region there are both anastomoses between right and left sides and also in the head region between the catchment area of individual lymph node groups (temporal, submandibular lymph nodes).

## h) Drainage of the Lymph-Obligatory Load from the Brain

With the exception of some areas, the capillaries of the brain have
an essentially thicker basal membrane than in the rest of the body.
The nutrition of the ganglion cells here is via the glia cells rather than
by diffusion through the capillary wall. The glia cell takes from the
capillary nutrients important for the ganglion cell and supplies it with
them. The metabolic products take the reverse route from cell to capillary via the glia cell. Therefore no lymph-obligatory load should
accumulate in these areas. However there are regions in the brain
where the blood capillaries do not have this thick basal membrane.
To a certain extent the capillaries of these regions even have endothelial cells with openings. Above all these are areas in which hormones
or similar substances are produced [2]: the area of Area Postrema (on
the floor of the 4th ventricle), paraphysis, wall of the optic recess (on
the floor of the 3rd ventricle in front of the exit of the optic nerve),
Emminentia saccularis of the hypophyseal stalk, neurohypophysis
(very strongly vascularised), pineal body (on the roof and towards the
beginning of the 3rd ventricle).

For a long time it was suspected that the lymph-obligatory load
from the brain and especially these areas, drained via the cerebrospinal fluid. And this is partly true. It was established that a connection must exist between cerebrospinal fluid and the lymph nodes of
the neck. India ink or dyes, which behave like lymph-obligatory load,
were injected into the fluid. Thus it was possible to follow the path
taken by the ink and see in which lymph nodes it was to be found. It
was discovered in several places, namely those where particular brain
nerves leave the meninges and come out of the bony skull. Likewise,
it was found in the wall of arteries and veins in the brain, and in the
lymph vessels and lymph nodes of the neck. The path of the ink and
therefore the lymph-obligatory load could be followed precisely
along the Fila olfactoria (olfactory nerves). An ARACHNOIDEAL
SHEATH (arachnoidea = arachnoid membrane of the soft meninges) accompanies the Fila olfactoria where it goes through the
ethmoid bone, i.e. leaves the base of the skull. This sheath continues
into the perineurium of the nerves (perineurium = a loose connective
tissue surrounding the peripheral nerves). The injected ink was found
in great quantities in this arachnoidal sheath and in the perineurium.

Further, the histological picture shows numerous lymph vessels and lymph capillaries in and around the perineurium which also had ink in their lumen (Fig. 8, 9, 10).

It is calculated that approx. 40% of the lymph-obligatory load from the brain seeps along the arachnoid sheath of the OLFAC-TORY NERVES into the perineurium of the nerves. From there it is taken up by the numerous lymph capillaries existing in the nasal and palate mucous membranes. The situation on the arachnoid sheath of the optic nerve is similar. There too the prelymph can seep into the

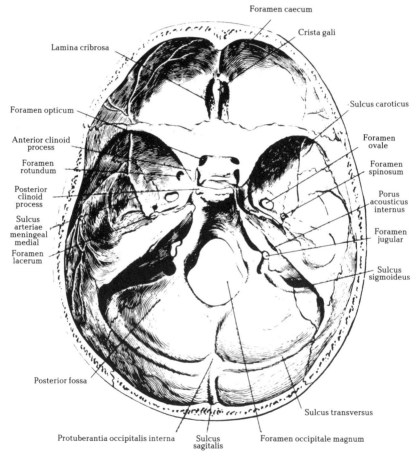

Fig. 8: Base of the skull. Inner surface *(Tandler*[26])

perineurium of the optic nerve with the fluid and be taken up by the numerous lymph capillaries in the retrobulbar tissue.

Many lymph capillaries lie in the jugular foramen, within the Dura mater and they drain through the jugular foramen to the jugular lymph trunks. The lymph-obligatory load of the Medulla oblongata (extended medulla) leaves the Foramen occipitale via the epidural lymph capillaries and is drained to the occipital lymph nodes.

A flow of prelymphatic fluid proceeds in the wall of the blood vessels of the brain and this can be traced right into the basal membrane of the brain capillaries. The stream of prelymph from the brain moves in these VIRCHOW-ROBIN intra adventitial spaces. Everywhere

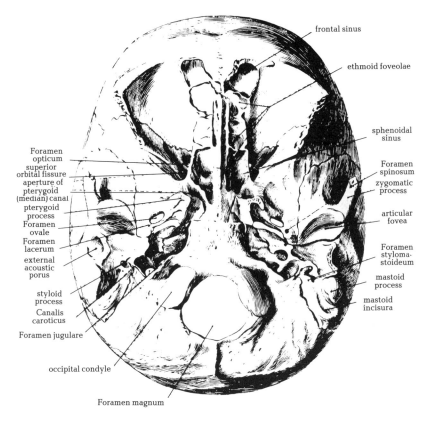

Fig. 9: [26])

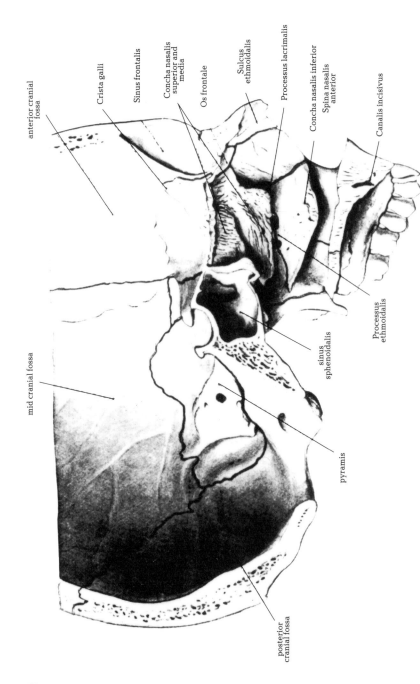

anterior cranial fossa

Crista galli

Sinus frontalis

Concha nasalis superior and media

Os frontale

Sulcus ethmoidalis

Processus lacrimalis

Concha nasalis inferior

Spina nasalis anterior

Canalis incisivus

Processus ethmoidalis

sinus sphenoidalis

mid cranial fossa

pyramis

posterior cranial fossa

Fig. 10: Median section through the skull. Sideview of the nasal cavity wall (*Tandler* [26])

vessels leave the skull, a great quantity of lymph capillaries is to be found in the walls of these vessels and in their surrounding tissues. As the vessel proceeds, these capillaries accept the prelymph from the VIRCHOW-ROBIN spaces.

Prelymph leaves the bony skull in the walls of the CAROTID ARTERY, JUGULAR VEIN, VEIN PLEXUS in the OCCIPITAL FORAMEN and the EMISSARY VEINS that leave the vault of the cranium.

Of the lymph that drains as prelymph along the Fila olfactoria through the ethmoid bone into the mucous membrane of the nasal and pharyngeal cavities and the palate, most is reached with inner mouth drainage.

The eye has lymph capillaries in the conjunctiva, eye muscles and retrobulbar fat tissue. Lymph-obligatory-load diffuses along the TENON capsule to the retrobulbar lymph vessels. The retrobulbar and conjunctiva lymph vessels are connected. [1] Perivascular (intra-adventitial) spaces have been traced in the retinal, opthalmic and internal carotid arteries and the arterial Circle of Willis. These are drained to the deep cervical lymph nodes. [8]

### i) Drainage of the Lymph-Obligatory Load from the Spinal Cord

The prelymph of the spinal cord leaves the spinal canal in the arachnoidal sheath of the spinal nerves (predominantly in the region of the lumbosacral plexus) (Fig. 11). The lymph capillaries appear as early as the epidural tissue. The arteries and veins in the spinal cord also have prelymphatic spaces in their walls which are drained via the spinal artery and vein to the paravertebral lymph vessels. The spinal canal can thus be drained with intensive paravertebral M.L.D. therapy.

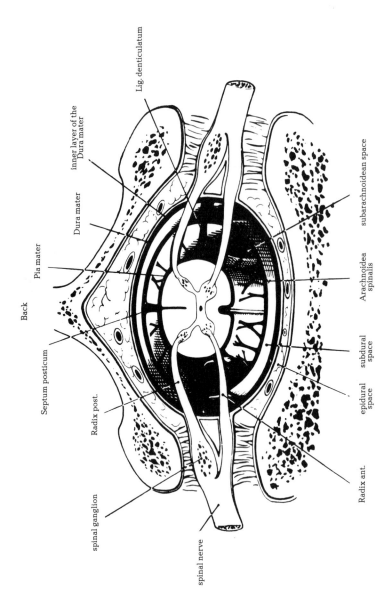

Lig. denticulatum

inner layer of the Dura mater

Dura mater

Pia mater

Back

Septum posticum

Radix post.

spinal ganglion

spinal nerve

subarachnoidean space

Arachnoidea spinalis

subdural space

epidural space

Radix ant.

Fig. 11: Cross section through the spinal column. Exit of the spinal nerves, position of the meninges. Vein plexus in epidural fat tissue. (*Corning* [27])

## 2. Structure of the Lymph Pathways

### a) Lymph Capillary [1, 3, 4]

The lymph capillary is the start of the lymphatic system. It lies in the interstitial tissue like the fingers of a glove, closed at one end. In many organs, the heart for example, the capillaries form a network. The capillary wall consists of a single ENDOTHELIAL CELL LAYER. These endothelial cells are connected in certain places with Zonulae adhaerens (relatively fixed connections). The free borders of the endothelial cells overlap and can move there like "SWINGING FLAPS". They are described as FLAP VALVES, because they can move outwards as well as inwards. The lymph capillary has no basal membrane. The endothelial cells are anchored with FILAMENTS to the collagen fibres of the connective tissue. These filaments are made of the same material as the collagen fibres. They also contain hyaluronic acid as a bonding substance.

A pair of LOBED VALVES lie between the lymph capillary and the adjoining lymph angion. Should fluid enter the ground substance of the connective tissue, it spreads out between the collagen fibres. Thus, the collagen fibres are pushed apart and take with them the endothelial cells by means of filaments attached to them. The flap valves are thus opened and the lymph-obligatory load pours into the lymph capillary from the tissue. When the capillary is full, the flap valves can close because of the pressure difference between inside and outside. The lobed valve opens and lymph flows into the adjacent lymph angion. Increased pressure in the area surrounding the lymph capillary can occur through muscle contraction or arterial pulse. The lymph capillary wall is not sealed and the small-molecular portion of lymph can diffuse back into the surrounding tissue. However the colloid-osmotic pressure difference arising because of this probably also plays a role in filling and emptying of the capillary. Also displacements in the gel-sol balance of the ground substance might also play a role here at the capillary. Lymph capillaries are larger than blood capillaries with a diameter between $20-60$ μm. Their length varies greatly (Fig. 12, 13).

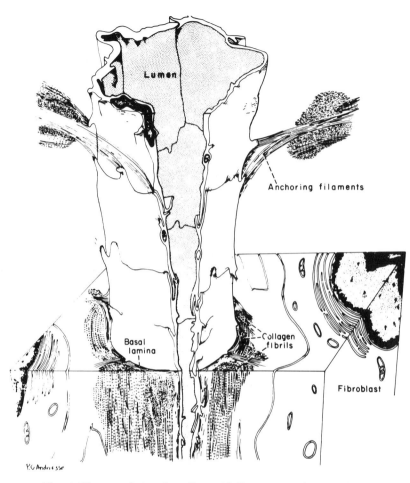

Fig. 12: Diagram of a lymph capillary with filaments *(Leak* and *Burke* [6])

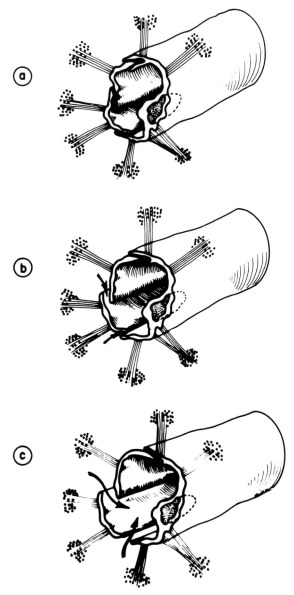

Fig. 13: Opening mechanism of the lymph capillary (*Leak* [6])

## b) Lymph Angions

The lymph angion is joined to the lymph capillary. Each angion extends from one lobed valve to the next and is a functional unit. The lymph angions strung together produce the lymph vessel. Under the microscope, they appear like a string of pearls: the muscle bellies out and then is constricted at the valves. The lobed valve is a double endothelial layer. The lymph angion has an ENDOTHELIAL CELL LAYER facing the lumen. Larger vessels have a mostly incomplete basal membrane, which is however more permeable than that of the blood capillaries. Smooth muscle cells arranged in a circle lie around the endothelial cell layer. The valve region is free of musculature. Numerous NERVE ENDINGS are found in the MUSCULATURE, from medullated and non-medullated nerves and with various types of endings: free ending, plexus or Father *Paccin* endings. The number of nerve endings suggests that each muscle cell is supplied by an axon. [5] Most of the axons are connected with the autonomic nervous system.

The musculature has an automatic autochthonicity (AUTO-MOTORICITY). [7] Characteristic electrical potentials are detected in an electro-lymphogram, and they also exist as a resting potential without muscle contraction. Their frequency varies between 5 — 10 potentials per minute. This also corresponds to the rhythm of muscle contractions without particular strain. Muscle contraction of the angions occurs quickly, whereas relaxation is slower. Neighbouring angions pulsate metachronously or in alternation. However they can also function with varying frequency and then there is invariably a pronounced co-ordination of the movement of neighbouring lymph angions. The influence on neighbouring lymph angions can occur from distal to proximal as well as from proximal to distal. The frequency of the lymph angion adapts itself to its content level: i.e., there is INCREASED FREQUENCY during LARGER LYMPH VOLUME. The increased frequency of a lymph angion can cause an increase of the frequency not only in the neighbouring lymph angion, but also in more remote lymph angion chains. This is of great significance for the effect of M.L.D. Through M.L.D. the motoricity of the lymph angion is stimulated not only in the area treated, but also in neighbouring zones.

An increase of the filling pressure raises the frequency and amplitude of the muscle contractions. STRETCH RECEPTORS in the lymph angion wall trigger this increased motoricity via REFLEX PATHWAYS over the spinal cord (see reflex). However, these reflex pathways should also run via peripheral autonomic ganglia near or in the lymph angion wall of larger vessels. Furthermore, a spontaneous form of excitation (automatic myogenic) should also occur in the musculature of the vessel wall (stretching of a muscle fibre leads to spontaneous contraction).

A raised inner pressure is not the only factor increasing lymph vessel motoricity. Crosswise and lengthwise stretching also have the same effect, as in the circular hand movements of the VODDER technique. However the effect of shearing forces can lead to spasms of the lymph vessels and thus hinder the lymph flow. Summarizing, one can say that light pressure in the vicinity of the vessel stimulates the lymph motoricity (e.g. the pulse of neighbouring arteries).

Likewise an INCREASE in TEMPERATURE causes an increased lymph motoricity. There are however limits to the effect of temperature on an increased frequency: above a maximum at 41 °C the frequency falls rapidly and eventually the motoricity comes to an irreversible halt. Cooling below 22 °C also brings the lymph vessel pulse to an irreversible halt. There is however an adaptation to cold, so that vessels initially held at below normal body temperature could be cooled more before the motoricity ceased because of cold.

The lymph vessel motoricity is controlled by the autonomic system. Just like histamine, adrenergic and cholinergic substances have a strong effect on the vessels. As far as the lymph is concerned, lactic acid ("aching muscles") and calcium effect an increase on the lymph motoricity, whereas the metabolites have no influence. [7] Faradic current produces spasms of the vessel. For a short while the frequency of the lymph motoricity can more than double. However a recovery phase then follows with decreased frequency.


### c) Large Lymph Trunks


The large lymph trunks have a similar wall structure to the veins, although the walls are thinner. The inner layer is formed of endothelial cells and after this comes an Elastica interna of collagen and elastic fibres. The muscularis has several layers in the large lymph trunks: inside there are two crossed, diagonal muscle spirals; in between there can be muscle fibres arranged in circles and longitudinal fibres can also be found under the adventitia in lymph vessels of the extremities. Frequently, stronger muscle fibres lie near the valves under the intima. The valve region itself is free of muscle. The vessel is wrapped in an adventitia through which nutrient vessels penetrate as far as the muscle layer. Smaller vessels also nourish their muscularis through diffusion from the vessel lumen. [5]

### d) Lymph Nodes (Fig. 14)

STRUCTURE: on its way through the lymph vessels, lymph passes through several lymph nodes. The regional lymph nodes lie near organs. The collector lymph nodes receive their supply from many large lymph vessels.

A lymph node can be anywhere from the size of a pin head to that of a bean. Inflammed lymph nodes can be significantly larger. The lymph node is bean-shaped and is dented in one place, the HILUM (stem). It has a CONNECTIVE TISSUE CAPSULE and septa, the trabeculae, which penetrate inside the lymph node giving it a framework.

Several lymph vessels join at the capsule although only 1 or 2 vessels leave the lymph node at the hilum. Also at this point, an artery enters and the vein leaves the lymph node. The blood vessels branch out in the trabeculae and pass through the lymph nodes with a thick capillary network. Underneath the capsule is a space filled with lymph, the MARGINAL SINUS, into which the endothelial cells (marginal cells) project. It continues along the trabeculae into the INTERMEDIARY SINUS. Inside the lymph node towards the hilum is the MEDULLARY SINUS Lymph flows into the marginal sinus in the supply vessels (AFFERENT LYMPH PATHWAYS). It flows through the intermediary sinus to the medullary sinus and leaves the lymph nodes by way of the EFFERENT PATHWAYS.

The basic framework of the lymph nodes between the trabeculae consists of RETICULAR TISSUE. Lymphocytes, macrophages and

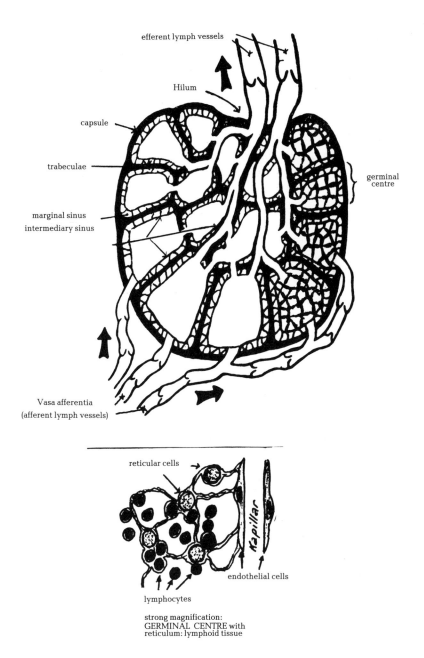

efferent lymph vessels

Hilum

capsule

trabeculae

germinal
centre

marginal sinus
intermediary sinus

Vasa afferentia
(afferent lymph vessels)

reticular cells

Kapillar

endothelial cells

lymphocytes

strong magnification:
GERMINAL CENTRE with
reticulum: lymphoid tissue

Fig. 14: Diagram of the lymph node (*Vodder* [25])

plasma cells are stored in this framework (reticular cells are also included as macrophages). The marginal cells occur in the marginal sinus and are special macrophages of the lymph nodes. Not only can they phagocytose, but they also play a role in antigen recognition (see immunology). Masses of lymphocytes lie under the marginal sinus in reticular tissue: the LYMPH FOLLICLE. These lymphocytes belong to the B series of lymphocytes and as long as they are characterized but not yet sensitised, we speak of a primary follicle. However if they are sensitized and contain germinal centres, they are known as secondary follicles. The germinal centres are in the middle of these follicles. Under the microscope they appear lighter than the other follicles. They contain lymphoblasts, the "mother cells" of the lymphocytes. To the side of the intermediary sinus (PARACORTICAL) are the lymphocytes of the T series. These T-lymphocytes can travel through the venioles in the blood system. This is known as the "recirculation of the lymphocytes". Along the vessels in the medullary sinus are the medullary funicles (filaments), which lead to the hilum. They contain numerous plasma cells which give up the content of their vesicle — gamma globulins — in the lymph vessels. Function of the lymph node:

1. it is a biological filter station.
2. approx. 40 % of the lymph-obligatory water load is resorbed here.
3. formation site for lymphocytes.
4. in connection with this, a function in the immunological system.

ad 1. Foreign substances such as dust or soot (pneumoconiosis with dust storage in the hilum of the lymph node) are filtered out of the lymph in the lymph node. Bacteria, cell debris and cancer cells are removed from the lymph vessel and held here. (Immunological defence against bacteria and cancer metastasis.) Infections can spread along the lymph vessels.

ad 2. Thickening of the lymph. If resorption is stronger than filtration at the blood capillaries in the lymph nodes, the surplus resorption force can draw fluid into the blood stream from the lymph saturated nodes. Therefore a greater volume of lymph flows in rather than out of the lymph nodes (more afferent than efferent vessels).

ad 3. Lymphocytes are formed in the lymph follicles and paracortical regions.

ad 4. These have an immunological function.

# 3. Lymph-Obligatory Load

According to *Földi* [3] lymph-obligatory load is described as the sum of various proteins and fluid as well as living and non-living particulate elements, which must be taken away by the lymph capillaries because they can no longer be taken up in the blood capillaries.

Thus the following are considered lymph-obligatory load:
1. plasma proteins — "protein load"
2. fluid — "water load"
3. non-auto-mobile cells — "cell load"
4. foreign substances
5. long chain fatty acids

ad 1. Plasma proteins reaching the tissues through micropinocytosis from blood capillaries can also be broken down by macrophages in the connective tissue (histiocytes). However this only applies to a fraction of the proteins. All other plasma proteins must be carried away via the lymph vessels. Hormones and enzymes bound to protein are also considered lymph-obligatory, as are lipoproteins.

ad 2. Fluid. If filtration forces exceed resorption forces at the capillaries, the fluid in the tissue is thus lymph-obligatory load.

ad 3. Non-auto-mobile cells. Erythrocytes, cell debris, dead cells, cells which have lost their cell groups (such as cancer cells), micro- and macrophages with phagocytosed contents (dead cells) all belong to this group. Erythrocytes are not auto-mobile cells and therefore must be taken away as lymph-obligatory load, via the lymph system, as soon as they have left the blood stream. If cancer cells are taken to the lymph nodes and multiply there, metastases develop.

ad 4. Foreign substances. Particulate substances like soot, dust, bacteria, dyes such as those used to show the lymph pathways.

ad 5. Long chain fatty acids which are reabsorbed from the chyme in the intestine must be taken away by the intestinal lymph. (Short chain fatty acids are transported via the portal venous system.) The amount of intestinal lymph can be reduced through a diet rich in short-chain fatty acids. [2]

# 4. Lymph

What is meant by lymph?
The contents of the lymph vessel are called lymph. The lymph-obligatory load is, of course, included here. Furthermore the contents are similar to those of the blood plasma, and have similar components: electrolytes and nonelectrolytes. The protein content, also part of the lymph-obligatory load, varies in the lymph in different parts of the body. Lymph can coagulate because it contains fibrinogen (a protein). In terms of cells, lymphocytes are found above all others in the lymph. Granulocytes are found there also. The concentration of lymphocytes varies in different sections of the lymph vessel. The lymph in the large lymph trunks contains more lymphocytes. Likewise, they are increased during inflammatory processes.

Lymph fluid is lost along the course of the lymph vessels because their walls are permeable to fluid. In addition, lymph fluid is withdrawn from the nutrient capillaries in the lymph vessel wall through resorption on the venous capillary loop.

# 5. Prelymph

Prelymph is described as lymph-obligatory load as long as it is still in the tissue and not yet in the lymph vessels. Numerous prelymphatic pathways are also found in the blood vessel wall, especially on the inner side of the skull. [2] Prelymphatic streams can increase in the walls of blood vessels in those parts of the body where the lymph vessels are not fully operative.

# 6. Lymph Volume

The volume of the lymph depends on the structure of the blood capillaries in the respective organs and on their circulation. If, during warm weather, the blood capillary network is dilated to regulate temperature balance, the filtration at these capillaries increases. During physical exertion — large nutrient requirement — the blood capillaries are dilated. The *Starling* equilibrium shifts in favour of an increased filtration and therefore a great lymph-obligatory load accumulates. Likewise, the volume of lymph increases in the digestive organs after intake of nutrients. More lymph-obligatory load occurs in the musculature during muscle work. Lymph is continually produced in organs which are constantly active (heart, lungs, glands with inner secretions). Approx. 2 litres of lymph flow through the mouth of the thoracic duct within 24 hours. The volume of lymph increases during warmth and is low during cold. During sleep, lymph-obligatory load comes only from those organs which are active during sleep.

# 7. Lymph Flow

Lymph flow comes about through:
1. The motoricity of the lymph angion
   a) auto-motoricity of the angion
   b) reflex action of the motoricity intensified by stretch stimulation
2. Effect of pressure and tension on the lymph vessel
   a) pulsation of neighbouring arteries
   b) contraction of neighbouring skeletal musculature
   c) manual lymph drainage
3. Abdominal breathing. Through the fall in intra-thoracic pressure during diaphragmatic breathing, suction is applied to the intake area of the thoracic duct. Lymph is thus sucked from the abdominal part of the thoracic duct to the thoracic section. This suction also encourages the lymph flowing into the venous arch. Thus, in therapy, one can favourably influence both lymph flow into the thoracic duct through abdominal breathing and also lymph flow at the confluence in the venous arch through appropriate breathing therapy, e.g. stretch-positioning exercises.

What promotes lymph flow?

Exertion and warmth promote lymph flow whereas cold hinders it. Venous stasis of the legs increases the lymph volume. Tight clothing can hinder lymph drainage. Because muscle activity increases lymph flow and promotes transportation in the venous system so that less lymph-obligatory load arises, lack of exercise and possibly even sedentary occupations increase the supply of lymph-obligatory load.

According to *Földi* the function of the lymph system can be briefly summarized as follows: safety valve function during disruption of the *Starling* equilibrium, extravascular circulation of plasma proteins and lipids, transportation of particulate elements from the interstitium. [2]

# D) Effect of Manual Lymph Drainage on the Nervous System

## 1. Effect of M.L.D. on the Autonomic Nervous System

Manual lymph drainage has a calming effect. This effect on the autonomic nervous system can be explained as a CHANGE FROM A SYMPATHETIC to a PARASYMPATHETIC STATE and through the triggering of ATTRACTION REFLEXES. It is important that the M.L.D. technique is carried out evenly for this change to occur and to elicit the attraction reflex: circular motions with a steady increase and decrease of pressure, with the correct degree of pressure (too great a pressure leads to a release of histamine in the tissue with hyperaemia and pain sensation) and with an even rhythm so that the stimulation can elicit an attraction reflex (see reflex).

However the comfort of the treatment room should not be overlooked: correct room temperature and covering of the untreated parts of the body, no excessive noise (constant radio playing), the lighting should not dazzle the patient. What about conversations between the therapist and the patient during treatment? During M.L.D. the patient should be able to relax fully and "accept" the therapy. If I involve her/him in an interesting discussion, the relaxation is hindered. But if it is a patient who likes to talk, to 'unburden' her/himself, then this aids relaxation. However these conversations should be "restful" without argument. If the tension has abated, the patient will be quiet because she/he has relaxed.

## 2. Analgesic Effect of M.L.D. [10]

In order to understand the analgesic effect of M.L.D. I would like to explain some basic concepts:

### a) Ganglion Cell, Glia Cell (Fig. 15)

The ganglion cell is the organ cell of the central nervous system (CNS). In addition there are various types of glia cells involved in the structure of the CNS. The glia cells form the support tissue of the CNS. Also they take care of the nutrition of the ganglion cell. On one side, with their extensions, they surround the blood capillaries, which have a very thick basal membrane in the brain. On the other side they surround the ganglion cells. Through an active process ("pumping"), they take out nutrients from the blood stream and carry them through their cell body to the ganglion cell. In the reverse direction, the metabolic products are taken from the cell. The glia cell does not accept all the substances provided in the blood for the ganglion cell but makes a choice. We speak of the blood-brain barrier, that is, not all substances present in the blood, e.g. medicines, reach the ganglion cell in the same concentration.

The EXCITATION PATHWAY occurs via the ganglion cell. This cell consists of cell membrane, protoplasm and a nucleus; it has numerous mitochondria (this means that energy-rich metabolic processes occur), endoplasmic reticulum (protein synthesis), Golgi apparatus, one or two long extensions (NEURITES) and many various short extensions (DENDRITES). Several neurites are bundled together to form peripheral nerves. The medullated nerves have a myelin sheath. In addition there are poorly medullated and non-medullated nerves. The conduction velocity in a neurite is decided by its thickness and whether or not it is medullated. Medullated, thick neurites have the greatest conduction velocity. [22]

Here are some measurements which illustrate the order of magnitude in which diameter and conduction velocity vary. [22]

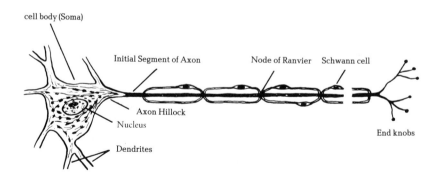

Fig. 15: Diagram of ganglion cell. Motor neurone with myelinised axon (*Ganong* [22])

| | diameter | conduction velocity |
|---|---|---|
| medullated neurites | 3 – 20 μm | up to 120 m/s |
| partly medullated neurites | up to 3 μm | 15 m/s |
| non-medullated neurites | up to 1 μm | 2 m/s |

The motor and sensory pathways consist of medullated neurites, whereas the pain pathways have non-medullated neurites.

Conduction in the neurites always occurs in one direction only. The sensory nerves have a RECEPTOR at their beginning in the periphery; this percieves the stimulus and guides it along to the ganglion cell as an excitation. A synapse lies near the ganglion cell. The motor ganglion cell belonging to the peripheral nerves is in the anterior horn of the spinal cord. Conduction to the motor end plate ( = transmission point from neurite to muscle) occurs in its neurites. The nerve pathways consist of neurites and ganglion cells connected consecutively.

The excitation occurring via a nerve is an electrical process (action potential). This is converted to a chemical, then back to an electrical process in the synapse. Synapses also occur in the C.N.S. and the action potential is transmitted here in a direct electrical manner from neurite to ganglion cell.

## b) Structure of the Synapse [22]

The end of the neurite is distended to a knob shape. The cell membrane there is called the presynaptic membrane. The SYNAPTIC GAP lies under this knob, and just under the gap is the next ganglion cell (or dentrite) with its subsynaptic membrane. This continues into the postsynaptic membrane. Various carrier substances occur at the synapses. Initially the mechanism was investigated at synapses with acetylcholine as a carrier substance. The neuromuscular, parasympathetic (pre- and postganglion) and sympathetic preganglion synapses have acetylcholine as a carrier substance (TRANSMITTER).

Noradrenalin is the transmitter in sympathetic postganglion synapses. In addition dopamine and serotonin are known to be carrier substances at the synapses of the CNS.

The mechanism of excitation transmission at synapses is known to have acetylcholine as a transmitter. Numerous mitochondria are found in the synapse foot (small knob), which means that much energy is used here. Also, there are many VESICLES in the synapse foot which contain carrier substance, in this case acetylcholine. If an excitation comes to the synapse in the form of an electrical potential, the vesicles move through the presynaptic membrane into the synaptic gap. Acetylcholine pours into the gap. The presence of acetylcholine causes a depolarization (through a massive influx of sodium ions) at the subsynaptic membrane. This means that an excitation proceeds along the ganglion cells. The acetylcholine must be broken down immediately in the synaptic gap and this occurs through an enzyme, acetylcholine esterase. Its components, acetate and choline, are taken back into the synapse foot through the presynaptic membrane. Somewhat further along the axon, and with the assistance of choline acetylase, these two components are converted back into acetylcholine and stored in the vesicles in the synapse foot.

When this process is finished, the synapse can transmit impulses again. This refractory period lasts approx. 0.5 msec (thousandth of a second). If numerous synapses interrupt the nerve paths, the transmission of the stimulus takes correspondingly longer due to the refractory period of the synapses. Most ganglion cells have very many synapses. There are between one and over 5 000 synapses at the motor anterior horn ganglion cell.

The transmission to the individual synapses can be described locally as well as chronologically. Apart from the EXCITATORY SYNAPSES described already, there are also INHIBITORY SYNAPSES. They have a different excitatory substance which changes the negative charge of the ganglion cell membrane (e.g. in the form of a hyperpolarization). Thus an action potential arriving at this cell is subliminal, and therefore its further transmission is inhibited. This inhibitory mechanism is explained very simply here. It plays a large role in the pain-inhibitory effect of M.L.D. The inhibitory synapses sort and co-ordinate the numerous impulses, which affect the C.N.S. simultaneously, and which lead to excitation. Tetanus toxin, as well as strychnine, switches off the effect of the inhibitory synapses in the brain (by blocking them). Then every stimulus is answered and a reaction is set off in the effector organ (e.g. muscle). This leads to every light or sound stimulus causing a muscle contraction response.

Transmission at the synapses is always in the same direction. The direction of the reflex path in the reflex arc is thus given.

## c) Reflex Arc (Fig. 16)

A simple reflex arc consists of 2 nerve cells with their neurones. A receptor lies at the beginning of the afferent neuron (leading towards the body), which passes on the effecting stimulus as an excitation (electrical action potential). The ganglion cell of this neuron mostly lies in the spinal ganglion and has a synapse to a motor anterior horn ganglion cell. The excitation is passed on from there via the efferent neuron to a motor end-plate at a muscle cell and triggers a contraction. These simple, monosynaptic reflex arcs occur with tendon reflexes (e.g. the patellar reflex, where stretching the patellar tendon results in contraction of the quadriceps femoris muscle). This is also an example of an autoreflex where the receptor and effector organ are in the same organ. Polysynaptic reflexes (reflex arcs via several synapses) and heterogenous reflexes (receptor and effector organ not in the same organ) are much more common.

In the animal kingdom, reflex actions are important protective mechanisms. This also applies to humans. Reflexes happen very quickly and unconsciously (without cerebral influence). The switching centre lies in the spinal cord. The reflex proceeds according to a predetermined pattern. Flight reflexes, which can be triggered through pain, proceed reflexively, and so do many reactions concerning the balance.

If the reflex is triggered by a strong pain, it can jump to other segments in the spinal cord. The autonomic nervous system can also participate: in cases of intense pain, the skin becomes pale, sweat comes out of the pores and even a collapse can occur.

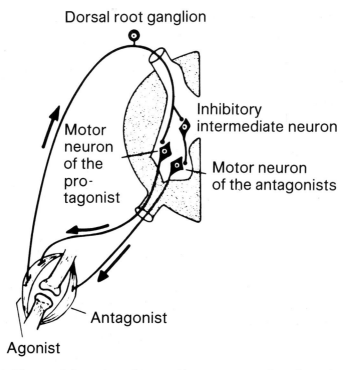

Dorsal root ganglion

Motor
neuron
of the
pro-
tagonist

Inhibitory
intermediate neuron

Motor neuron
of the antagonists

Antagonist

Agonist

Fig. 16: Diagram of the tendon reflex arc with a sensory nerve from the tendon spin-
dle, sensory ganglion cell, connection with excitatory synapse of the extensor and with
inhibitory synapse of the flexor. (*Ganong* [22])

### d) Attraction Reflex

Both the attraction and withdrawal reflexes can be elicited in a frog
preparation where the connection between the spinal cord and the
higher centres of the C.N.S. have been interrupted. [10] If the frog's
foot is stroked with a cold, smooth, damp finger, the foot moves
towards the stroking. This is an attraction reflex. Similarly, the clasp-
ing reflex of the male frog is an attraction reflex, which however is
connected with a flexion of the front feet. Not every attraction reflex
is associated with extension, nor is every flight reflex connected with
flexion. The form of the stimulus is decisive as to whether an attraction or withdrawal reflex is elicited. This says something about the

characteristics of the stimulus. If we want to elicit an attraction reflex with M.L.D., then the stimulus created by the massage must be appropriate: the therapist's hands should be pleasantly warm; the pressure should produce neither friction nor pain; the movements should be delivered evenly and rhythmically. An attraction reflex is more difficult to trigger than a withdrawal reflex. If different stimuli have a simultaneous effect, thus causing an attraction reflex on the one hand and a withdrawal reflex on the other, or if several stimuli have a simultaneous effect which can release both attraction and withdrawal reflexes, then the stronger stimulus will be the effective one up to a point. The withdrawal reflex predominates with stimuli of equal strength.

### e) Mechanism of the Analgesic Effect of M.L.D. [10]

M.L.D. not only has a calming and relaxing effect, but also reduces pain. As long as there is pain, the pain receptors send their action potentials. These pain signals are passed through an intermediate connection in the spinal cord and via the brain stem to the cerebrum. When the pain is perceived as such in the cerebrum, we become aware of it. Then we can do something either to eliminate the cause of the pain or to take care of an injury.

The pain receptor fires action potentials as long as the pain lasts, according to the degree of pain. With M.L.D., the skin is stroked near the pain stimulus. Touch receptors in the skin perceive this stroking. However touch receptors are capable of sending action potentials only at the beginning and ending of contact. Therefore they merely register a change in the state of contact. Nerve fibres of the touch receptors have their switching stations in the spinal cord. The impulse goes from there to the cerebrum and registers the touch, which we then consciously perceive. However, in the spinal cord the nerve fibre has a colateral (lateral pathway) to an inhibitory cell. This inhibitory cell is connected to the switch-cell of the pain pathway. If the inhibitory cell receives an impulse, it passes this on as an inhibition. If the touch receptor registers a stimulus and conducts it as an impulse to the spinal cord, the inhibitory cell always transforms this impulse into an inhibition, and thus interrupts the transmission of

83

pain at the switch cell of the pain pathway in the spinal cord. If the touch receptor is touched once, an inhibition is produced. However with stroking, several neighbouring touch receptors are stroked in succession. Each of these receptors sends action potentials at the beginning and end of contact. Each of these action potentials causes an inhibition of the pain transmission. Therefore, with M.L.D., the "stroking" can cause a reduction in pain. This inhibitory effect on pain transmission does have a limit though. The inhibitory effect of the stroking movements are too weak to affect very strong pain.

The pain-relieving effect often plays a large role in the use of M.L.D. For example, with painful haematoma, swollen oedemas or *Sudeck's* dystrophy, it is possible to utilize fully the oedema-reducing effect of M.L.D. through this pain reduction for the first time.

# E) Effect of Manual Lymph Drainage on Skeletal and Vessel-Wall Musculature

# 1. Effect of Skeletal Musculature

A normalization of muscle tonus can be achieved in cases of hypertonus and aching muscles (accumulation of lactic acid indicating oxygen deficient metabolism). The lactic acid is drained via the lymph vessels, frequently in combination with applications of heat. Of course, the cause of the hypertonus must be sought and taken into consideration.

# 2. Effect on Musculature Wall of Lymph Vessel

M.L.D. stimulates the LYMPH MOTORICITY and leads to an increase in the TRANSPORT CAPACITY. The spasm of spastically narrowed lymph vessels (hypertonus) can be alleviated by M.L.D. The lymph motoricity is also stimulated in over-extended, congested lymph vessels. Both the frequency and amplitude of the contractions can be increased. The contraction stimulus can effect both the neighbouring and more distant lymph angions. We may assume that M.L.D. treatment of the neck works in this way on the lymph vessels joining the venous arch (thoracic duct and Ductus lympaticus dexter with lymph vessels leading into it).

# 3. Effect on Peristalsis

Experience shows that spastic constipation can be brought to a normal intestinal motility with M.L.D. treatment. The same is true for intestinal sluggishness with reduced tonus. The mechanism of intestinal MYOGENIC AUTONOMY suggests itself as an explanation: AUTORHYMICITY can be triggered by stretching of the intestinal muscle fibres. This stretching of the intestine causes a depolarization of the muscle cells with its resultant muscle contraction. With M.L.D., coordination of peristalsis occurs in the individual sections.

# F) Effect of Manual Lymph Drainage on the Defence System of the Body

The favourable effect of M.L.D. on the defence system of the body is known to us through experience. However this effect has yet to be proven scientifically. Therefore we can only offer it as an hypothesis based on experience. For exactly that reason, however, it seems to us important to understand the nature of the defence system and therefore to describe it in more detail.

We differentiate:
1. Non-specific defence system:
   a) cellular
      α) microphages
      β) macrophages
   b) humoral

2. Specific defence system = immunological defence system
   a) cellular
   b) humoral
   c) immune tolerance
   d) autoallergic illnesses
   e) homeostasis in the immune system


## 1. Non-Specific Defence System

### a) Cellular

Micro- and macrophages are understood to be cells that can destroy pathogens, foreign substances or dead cells through phagocytosis and intracellular enzymatic breakdown.


### α) Microphages

There are relatively small cells, the granulocytes of the blood (see blood). When they have destroyed foreign substances through phagocytosis, they perish. Then they are either eaten by macrophages or they leave the body as pus (dead granulocytes in liquid ground substance).

## β) Macrophages

Not only are these cells of the unspecific defence system but they also play a role in the specific defence system (they bind antigen, receive information and pass it on to the cells of the specific immune system). Their unspecific ability to phagocytose can be intensified by antigens.

They are summarized as the RHS SYSTEM (RETICULOHIS-TIOCYTIC SYSTEM). The RES = reticuloendothelial system belongs to this.

These cells have in common that they occur in connective or reticular tissue, they can phagocytose and can deliver immunological information to some extent. The RHS-system comprises:

| | |
|---|---|
| histiocytes | (mobile connective tissue cells, see connective tissue). |
| monocytes | (see blood). |
| marginal cells | macrophages of the lymph node sinus and bone marrow capillaries. |
| **Kupffer's** | stellate cells in the liver. |
| mesoglia cells | lie in brain tissue around the blood vessels. |
| reticular cells | phagocytic reticular cells which occur in reticular tissue, e.g. in lymph nodes. |
| adventitia cells | macrophages in the immediate vicinity of capillaries and venioles. |

## b) Humoral

This concerns substances (proteins) which are passed from the cells into the serum for non-specific defence against foreign substances. [13] This includes INTERFERON which is released from virus-infected cells and inhibits the multiplication of viruses in other cells. It is effective before the antibody reaction to the virus infection develops. PYROGENS (fever producing substances) can also be cited here. Bacterial and viral products work as exogenous pyrogens and cause endogenous pyrogens to form in micro- and macrophages. These have an effect on the temperature regulation centre in the hypothalamus and produce fever. Fever is an important factor in the fight against viruses.

# 2. Specific Defence System = Immunological Defence System

Certain foreign substances — frequently proteins but also carbohydrates and industrial chemical products — can have an ANTIGENIC property in the body. That is they stimulate the body to form ANTIBODY which is a specific, effective defence against them. The antibody is specific to this one antigen. Antigen and antibody fit together like lock and key. Once formed, this antibody adheres to a memory cell and causes the formation of a large amount of this antibody when the immune system is restimulated. They break down the infiltrating antigen so that no actual illness is produced: the body has become immune to this pathogen.

However the body can also form antibodies against substances that we come into contact with daily: detergent, cement, paint, grass pollen, cat hair, flour etc. If someone forms an antibody against one of these substances, each contact with this substance (antigen) can start a rapid ANTIGEN-ANTIBODY REACTION. We refer to an ALLERGY against any particular substance. Because these antibodies (Ig E) often adhere to mast cells, histamine can escape from the mast cell into the surrounding tissue during the antigen-antibody reaction. Thus this allergic reaction is characterized by the effects of histamine. On the skin: redness (dilation of the capillaries), oedema (increased permeability and blood pressure in the small vessels), local increase in temperature (opening of the arterial sphincters). In the bronchioles: bronchiole spasm, swelling of the mucous membrane (oedema). In the nose: local oedema of the nasal mucous membrane with increased secretion (rhinitis).

When surgeons first considered skin and then organ transplants, they needed initially to explain the circumstances under which a transplant would be accepted or rejected. This area of surgery therefore has made much progress in immunological research.

Lymphocytes and other cells of the lymphatic organs play a large role in both types of immunological reactions. CELLULAR IMMUNITY concerns the effective antibodies which adhere directly to a cell (lymphocyte) itself where they render the antigens harmless. HUMORAL IMMUNITY refers to antibodies given to the plasma from plasma cells. The course of the different immunological reactions depends on many factors. Macrophages and various cells of the lymphatic system make a supportive contribution. Therefore I should like to describe simply the basic principles of both types of immunological defence. [15]


### a) Cellular

Lymphocytes formed in the bone marrow still have no immunological capability whatsoever. Some of them migrate to the THYMUS to become IMMUNOLOGICALLY CHARACTERIZED there through a maturing process. These cells then move into the lymphatic tissue (lymph nodes, tonsils, spleen), stamped as T-lymphocytes. 'Stamped' means they are equipped to undertake a specific immunological function. 'T-lymphocytes' means they receive this characteristic in the thymus. They then lie in the paracortical areas in the lymph nodes. If an antigen enters the body, it can SENSITIZE these STAMPED T-LYMPHOCYTES. That is, it and all its 'followers' carry an antibody in or on their cells which is specific for this antigen. As soon as this lymphocyte is sensitized, it multiplies, thereby passing on to its daughter cells its specific ability to recognize and break down the antigen that sensitized it. The T-IMMUNOBLAST stage forms the T-IMMUNOCYTES (T-lymphocytes) which can now fight against all antigens of this type infiltrating the body.

One of these T-lymphocytes remains behind as a "memory". These MEMORY CELLS are long lived, up to one year. Afterwards, one of the daughter cells takes over this memory function. If the same antigen comes into the body again, it is recognized by this memory cell and multiplication proceeds via the T-immunoblast and T-immunocyte. The besieging antigens are broken down by the antibodies of the T-immunocytes, so that no signs of illness appear. The body is immune to this illness. With mumps and measles, IMMUNISATION proceeds according to this mechanism. It is T-lymphocytes that react in many viral infections, some bacterial illnesses, toxoplasmosis, transplant rejections, autoimmune illnesses, 'tumor supervision' in the body and in many allergies. T-lymphocytes can have a direct cell-destroying effect (cytotoxic). The function of other T-lymphocytes is to help B-lymphocytes during the humoral immulogical reaction. Others activate macrophages to phagocytose or release mediators (effective substances).

To a certain degree, the body has the ability to restrict excessive growth of degenerated cells — tumor growth — by means of the T-lymphocytes. The body can recognize cells that originally come from the body but are degenerated and multiplying with excessive speed. They are rendered harmless by the T-lymphocytes. Because of this, such excessive cell growth can be halted in a microscopic area. Tumor growth can take over because this defence mechanism is very susceptible to interference (e.g. through blockage of the place where the antigen binds to the lymphocyte). Spontaneous recovery from carcinomas can be affected by T-lymphocyte activity.

Generally, this fight against tumors is dependant on their size. They are difficult to detect with the present tumor search methods. If the tumor has escaped the control of the T-lymphocytes, it frequently grows undetected for a while longer. Of course it also depends on the location of the tumor, whether an early diagnosis can be made, for example through biopsy, or if we rely on the evidence of x-ray examination or scintigram.

### b) Humoral

Lymphocytes originating in bone marrow receive their STAMPING in the so called BURSA EQUIVALENT. In birds, the stamping is carried out in the Bursa fabricii. In humans there must be a corresponding organ to this bursa, where the B-lymphocytes are stamped. At present it is assumed that this could occur in the PEYERS patches of the intestine, the lymphatic ring of the pharynx or even in the bone marrow. The stamped B-lymphocytes settle in the lymph node follicles and the lymphocytic sheaths of the spleen. If stamped lymphocytes are in the follicles, we refer to a PRIMARY FOLLICLE. If they are already sensitized, they are in the SECONDARY FOLLICLES. The sensitization occurs likewise through contact with antigen. Inside the secondary follicles there are germinal centres with lymphoblasts. Numerous antibodies are carried on the surface of the sensitized lymphocytes and these are antigen-specific. Plasmablasts are formed in lymph nodes after the first contact with antigen. [16] These move into the medullary funicles and, as mature plasma cells, release immunoglobulin. In addition, the lymph follicles react by forming germinal centres. Through contact with the antigen, plasma cells are formed which release immunoglobulin, and also small lymphocytes are formed in the germinal centres. The small lymphocytes carry specific antibody on their surface. It is the B MEMORY CELLS that recognize antigen when there is renewed contact with antigen. They trigger the formation of immunoglobulins via the plasma cells.

B-lymphocytes can form antibodies after contact with antigen, but often need the additional help of macrophages or T-lymphocytes.

Not every immunity remains for an unlimited time. Some become weaker over the course of the years, although they can also be strengthened after re-exposure to antigen. The ability of the body to build up an immunological defence is used in immunization. In active immunization, the body is brought into contact with weakened, killed or related pathogens so that it can build antibodies ( = immunity) against the disease. A booster vaccination re-stimulates antibody formation through renewed contact with the antigen. In passive immunization, friendly gamma globulin specifically developed against this disease is injected into the body. Passive immunization lasts for a few weeks only.

Gamma globulins released from plasma cells are a component of plasma proteins. Five different gamma globulins are known: (Ig) A, D, E, G, M. Ig A formed from plasma cells is provided with its own factor from the mucous membrane cells and secreted, for example, on the surface of the respiratory tract mucous membrane. From there, this Ig A reaches the antigen even before it can penetrate the body through the mucous membrane. Ig A is also secreted from intestinal mucosa or secretory glands such as mammary glands or salivary glands. Ig M (for macro) is a large molecule. It is often formed first in a humoral reaction and then relieved by Ig G. Likewise, the rheumatoid factor of P.C.P. is an Ig M molecule. Ig G is the most common gamma globulin and has the highest concentration in plasma. It is responsible for many humoral immune reactions. Ig E only occurs in small amounts in the serum, although it plays a large role in allergic reactions (it was described earlier as reagin). It can adhere to mast cells and then histamine is released during the antigen-antibody reaction. Ig D is only contained in very small amounts in the serum.

### c) Immune Tolerance

Once in a while antibodies fail to form, although antigens are having an effect on the body. The inability to form antibodies against the antigen is described as tolerance. Tolerance can have various causes: congenital tolerance, acquired tolerance.

CONGENITAL TOLERANCE. The body recognizes its own protein, which was there at the time of birth. Under special circumstances the body can recognize its own tissue as "foreign" and form antibodies against it. We refer then to an AUTOALLERGIC ILLNESS. The body's tolerance to its own substances is broken down.

ACQUIRED TOLERANCE. Tolerance will develop: if antigens penetrate the body in large quantities; if insufficient contact with the microphages is achieved; if the antigens work in very small amounts at short intervals. Tolerance formation through repeated contact with very small amounts of antigen applies during the desensitization against allergens ( = substances that trigger allergies). In order to produce tolerance during organ transplants, anti-lymphocyte sera (antibody against the body's own lymphocytes), radiotherapy, cortisone and cytostatica (cell damaging substances) are used.

Tolerance also arises with a defective immune system: a thymus that has stopped working or lack of immunoglobulin fraction. Tolerance maintains itself through very small amounts of antigen. It is also specific.

### d) Autoallergic Illnesses

There are a series of autoallergic illnesses in which the body forms antibodies against its own components. More often than not, these substances were not in the body at birth, or developed into foreign substances through illness.

P.C.P.: autoallergy against the body's own antigenic synovial membrane which becomes "foreign" through inflammatory processes. As such the autoallergy is not treatable with M.L.D., although the chronic inflammatory symptoms of P.C.P. probably are.

LUPUS ERYTHEMATOSUS: autoallergy against nucleoproteins and D.N.A. of the cell nucleus. HASHIMOTO'S THYROIDITIS: autoallergy against the thyroid hormone. HAEMOLYTIC ANAEMIAS can be caused by autoimmune reactions. In MYASTHENIA GRAVIS, correlations with autoimmune processes are seen. MULTIPLE SCLEROSIS, too, is associated with autoimmune reactions. An autoallergic component can also be involved in ULCERATIVE COLITIS.

### e) Homeostasis in the Immune System

In the healthy body there is a balance (homeostasis) between immune response and tolerance. If the balance is disrupted in favour of the immune response, this can lead to allergies or autoimmune reactions. If the balance changes in favour of tolerance, an ANERGY (absence of the immune response) or malignant tumors (malignant systemic disease) can develop. [17] Intact lymphatic organs protect against a breakdown of the immunological system.

Our experience has demonstrated that Dr. *Vodder's* M.L.D. enables the body's defence system to react well. Because M.L.D. promotes lymph flow through lymph vessels and nodes, the antigens are brought more rapidly to the lymph nodes, where the antibodies can more quickly exercise their effect.

# Bibliography

[1] *Rusznyak, J., Földi, M.* und *Szabo, G.:* Lymphologie. Gustav Fischer Verlag. Stuttgart 1969.

[2] *Földi, M.:* Erkrankungen des Lymphgefäßsystems. Gerhard Witzstrock Verlag. Baden-Baden 1971.

[3] *Földi, M., Klücken, N.* und *Collard, M.:* Praxis der Lymphgefäß- und Venenerkrankungen. Gustav Fischer Verlag. Stuttgart 1974. Aus: Handbuch der allgemeinen Pathologie, 3. Bd., 6. Teil. Springer Verlag. Berlin-Heidelberg-New York 1972, folgende Arbeiten [4-7]:

[4] *Földi, M.:* Physiologie und Pathophysiologie des Lymphgefäßsystems.

[5] *Wenzel, J.:* Normale Anatomie des Lymphgefäßsystems.

[6] *Leak, L. V.:* The Fine Structure and Function of the Lymphatic Vascular System.

[7] *Mislin, H.:* Die Motorik der Lymphgefäße und die Regulation der Lymphherzen.

[8] *Grüntizig:* Referat auf der Arbeitstagung der Gesellschaft für Manuelle Lymphdrainage 1977.

[9] *Kuhnke:* Das Bindegewebe. Physiotherapie **64**, Heft 9.

[10] —: Der Schmerz als Reflex. Empfindung und Affekt. Physiotherapie **65**, Heft 4.

[11] —: Die physiologischen Grundlagen der ML. Physiotherapie **66**, Heft 12.

[12] *Pischinger, A.:* Das System der Grundregulation. 7., verb. Auflage, Karl F. Haug Verlag. Heidelberg 1989. Aus: *Vorlaender,* Praxis der Immunologie. Georg Thieme Verlag. Stuttgart 1976, folgende Arbeiten [13-17]:

[13] *Hahn, H.* und *Opferkuch, W.:* Mechanismen der immunologischen Infektabwehr.

[14] *Tilz, G. P.:* Folgereaktionen.

[15] *Resch, K.:* Zelluläre Immunreaktionen.

[16] *Kowatzki, E.:* Antigene und Antigenität/Humorale Immunreaktionen.

[17] *Götz, H.:* Tumorimmunologie.

[18] *Wendt, L.:* Krankheiten verminderter Kapillarmembranpermeabilität. Verlag E. E. Koch 1973 (mittlerweile als Nachdruck im Karl F. Haug Verlag erschienen).

[19] *Földi, E.:* Das Intervallstadium des Lymphödems — die Bedeutung der extralymphatischen zellularen Plasmaproteinbewältigung. Zeitschrift für Lymphologie I, 2 (1977) Schattauer Verlag. Stuttgart.

[20] *Casley-Smith, J. R.:* The Actions of the Benzo Pyrones on the Blood-Tissue-Lymph-System. Folia Angiologica 24, 1/2 (1976).

[21] *Siegenthaler, W.:* Klinische Pathophysiologie. Georg Thieme Verlag. Stuttgart 1973.

[22] *Ganong:* Lehrbuch der medizinischen Physiologie. Springer Verlag. Berlin-Heidelberg-New York 1974.

[23] *Rein-Schneider:* Einführung in die Physiologie des Menschen. Springer Verlag. Berlin-Heidelberg-New York 1971.

[24] *Sieglbauer, F.:* Lehrbuch der normalen Anatomie des Menschen. Urban & Schwarzenberg. München 1963.

[25] *Vodder, E.:* Die manuelle Lymphdrainage ad Modum Vodder. Schema über Lymphbahnen und Lymphknoten.

[26] *Tandler, J.:* Lehrbuch der systematischen Anatomie. F. C. Vogl. Leipzig 1926.

[27] *Corning, H. K.:* Lehrbuch der topographischen Anatomie. J. F. Bergmann, München 1919.

[28] *Tischendorf, F.:* Lymphatisches System. Demeter Verlag. Grafelfing 1980.

[29] *Tischendorf, F.* und *Földi, M.:* Die Berechnung des "optimalen Massagedruckes" — ein Mißbrauch der Starling-Formel. Physikalische Therapie in Theorie und Praxis 8/1981.